Quintessentials of Dental Practice – 21
Periodontology – 7

Contemporary Periodontal Surgery:

An Illustrated Guide to the Art Behind the Science

By

**Geoffrey Bateman, Shuva Saha,
Iain Chapple**

with contributions from
Craig Barclay and Chris Butterworth

Editor-in-Chief: Nairn H F Wilson
Editor Periodontology: Iain L C Chapple

D1356569

Quintessence Publishing Co. Ltd.

London, Berlin, Chicago, Paris, Milan, Barcelona, Istanbul,
São Paulo, Tokyo, New Delhi, Moscow, Prague, Warsaw

British Library Cataloguing in Publication Data

Contemporary periodontal surgery: an illustrated guide to the art behind the science.
- (Quintessentials of dental practice; v. 21)
1. Periodontics 2. Dentistry, Operative
I. Bateman, Geoffrey
617.6'32

ISBN-13: 9781850971238

ISBN-13: 978-1-85097-123-8

Foreword

Periodontal surgery; an integral element of the clinical practice of periodontology is both a science and an art. It spans a broad range of procedures involving the supporting tissues of the teeth, and has been extended in recent years to include soft tissue surgery in relation to dental implants. *Contemporary Periodontal Surgery: An Illustrated Guide to the Art behind the Science* concludes an excellent collection of volumes on periodontology in the *Quintessentials of Dental Practice* series. In common with all the other *Quintessentials* volumes on periodontology, let alone the other titles in the series, this book is an engaging, easy to read and extensively illustrated, authoritative overview of the subject area. If you have formed the view that surgery has little, if any, part to play in the modern clinical practice of periodontology, then it is especially important that you become familiar with this book, and use it, as intended, as a close-to-hand *aide memoire* in your clinical environment. The few hours it takes to read this volume will be time exceedingly well spent, with the prospect of you changing your clinical practice of surgical periodontology. If every picture says a thousand words, then this neat *Quintessentials*-sized volume is a deceptively small sized tome on periodontology; it is a veritable feast of valuable information of immediate practical relevance. Intrigued? Well, read on, enjoy and learn; this book – a scientific and artful text on modern periodontal surgery, will exceed your expectations.

Congratulations to the authors and editor on adding to the excellence of the *Quintessentials* series.

Nairn Wilson
Editor-in-Chief

Preface

Contemporary Periodontal Surgery is a book that aims to take the practitioner on a journey through the fundamentals of careful case selection and holistic pre-surgical planning, through the informed consent process and into the intricacies of periodontal microsurgery and post-surgical care, in an illustrated and stepwise manner. One of the key factors that differentiates periodontal surgery from other forms of oral surgery, is that the condition, shape and contours of the marginal and interproximal tissues post-surgery are fundamental outcome measures of the success of the operation. If a patient is unable to effect high standards of home care following periodontal surgery due to poor tissue contours, the surgery is likely to fail in the medium to longer term. Thus, delicate tissue management and attention to detail when closing surgical wounds is a prerequisite for success, as is the use of magnification, good field illumination and microsurgical instrumentation. These are a vital component of contemporary periodontal surgery.

One of the key paradigms which differentiates the best surgeon from the average surgeon is the working philosophy that "the feasibility of an operation is not an indication for its execution"; in other words, just because an operation is technically feasible does not mean that it is the correct thing to do for every patient in every situation. Competent surgeons think beyond the operation to its consequences and in particular the relative suitability of other approaches: sometimes the correct decision is the decision not to operate. A further consideration is that as a general guide, surgery has no place in the management of medical conditions; these require medical management, unless all medical options have failed. In this scenario, surgery is a last resort and as such should be contemplated with great caution.

This text therefore aims to provide the reader with a clear guide to planning periodontal surgery and an illustrated approach to the execution of a range of periodontal surgical procedures. The core principles underpinning treatment decisions and planning are discussed alongside the fundamentals of preparing the patient and the surgeon for the operation. A number of tips are provided to ensure patient comfort and the creation of an optimal operative field, thereby ensuring a smooth procedure, which minimises the risk of unforeseen events.

The techniques covered include resective procedures for diseased or unsightly tissues, mucoperiosteal flap access procedures and plastic surgery procedures designed to regenerate and replace lost or inflamed tissues. Finally, procedures executed to augment hard and soft tissues in preparation for implant placement are discussed.

Outcomes of Reading This Text

This text will not focus on the aetiology of lesions or conditions requiring surgical management; this is covered in earlier books in this series. It is hoped that having read this text the reader will be able to:

- Appreciate the alternative approaches to surgical intervention and when these may be more appropriate than the proposed surgery for a particular patient.
- Understand that managing medical conditions surgically is inadvisable and should only be contemplated as a last resort. Thus, no operation should be contemplated without a clear diagnosis, and clear surgical objectives that will benefit the patient.
- Understand the scope of periodontal surgery and the principles underpinning its safe practice.
- Appreciate the aims and objectives, indications and contraindications for periodontal surgery.
- Understand the impact of a patient's medical history upon the decision to operate or not.
- Understand and appreciate the need for and importance of informed consent.
- Appreciate the importance of sterile and aseptic technique.
- Understand the importance of and stages required for, pre-surgical and surgical planning.
- Be able to interpret the findings of routine clinical investigations (e.g. blood test results) and use these to inform their case planning.
- Be familiar with analgesic methods and those necessary to manage haemorrhage.
- Value and understand the tangible additional benefits of using appropriate magnification and field illumination.
- Appreciate the complications that may arise during an operation and immediately afterwards as well as in the medium and longer term.
- Have good knowledge of the principles of surgical flap design and execution as well as debridement and closure.
- Understand the differences between different flap compositions and designs and what may be most appropriate for different situations.

- Appreciate the importance of delicate handling of tissues and meticulous surgical technique to minimise tissue trauma.
- Advise their patient about immediate and longer term post-operative care.
- Identify their limitations and when to refer for advice or treatment by specialists.
- Be prepared to commit to regular review and re-appraisal of the patient and take long term responsibility for surgical outcomes.

Iain L C Chapple (ILC)

Chapter 1
Principles and Practice of Periodontal Surgery 1: Case Selection and Planning

Aim

The aim of this chapter is to provide the reader with a philosophy for case selection and treatment planning in periodontal surgery. Treatment objectives for predictable surgical management will be detailed alongside the principles common to different surgical procedures.

Outcome

Having read this chapter the reader will be able to carefully plan a surgical case and identify potential pitfalls on a case-by-case basis. The standardised evidence-based protocols described will help to enhance the operator's existing surgical preparation, irrespective of the type of surgery planned.

The Art and Science of Surgery

Periodontal surgery is both a science and an art. The periodontal surgeon should be both knowledgeable and ready to adapt their practice in line with the best research evidence. They should be able to critically appraise this evidence in an objective manner. In addition, the technical aspects of surgery require fine motor skills, gentle tissue handling and the visual anticipation of how a flap will close: this is the art of surgery. Surgical management requires a marriage of both of these facets, if excellence is to be achieved. Surgical skill comes through both didactic and observational learning, thorough experience and, to a lesser extent, the surgeon's innate dexterity. The importance of education, therefore, cannot be overstated.

The other key aspect of good surgical management is regular practice to guard against de-skilling. The practitioner should be ready to appraise their own abilities and not undertake cases beyond their limits of competence; these may change throughout the course of their career.

The archetypical Renaissance man, Leonardo da Vinci, was an example to modern-day surgeons. In his era, science and art were not regarded as mutually exclusive entities. His studies in science and engineering were as accomplished as his drawing and painting. Leonardo's drawing skills developed through his study of anatomy. A reproduction of one of his head and neck dissections may be found on the front cover of this text.

The Right Procedure

It is axiomatic that careful diagnosis and prescription of the right procedure are a *sine qua non* of surgical management. Future chapters will explore a selection of more popular surgical techniques and their indications in greater depth. The dental surgeon should be aware, however, of the nature and sequelae of the proposed treatment and be competent to carry out that treatment where appropriate. It follows that a full and frank discussion with the patient is necessary to gain informed consent. Informed consent should detail benefits, risks, other treatment options to be considered and what will happen if treatment is not carried out. Under common law, a conscious and competent patient needs to provide verbal consent to any operative procedure, although where sedation or deeper anaesthesia is employed, written consent is mandatory. Patients should also be provided with a written treatment plan and an estimate of costs.

The Right Patient

Appropriate patient selection is important if high success rates are to be achieved and maintained with surgery. There are few absolute contraindications to surgery in general dental practice.

Common contraindications include:
• severe bleeding diatheses
    – congenital, e.g. haemophilia and von Willebrand's disease
    – acquired, e.g. warfarinised patient with a high INR
      (international normalised ratio ≥ 3.5)
• significantly immunocompromised patients, e.g. acute leukaemia
• unstable angina
• poorly controlled diabetes
• uncontrolled hypertension.

With few exceptions, periodontal surgical procedures are elective in nature. All attempts should be made, therefore, to postpone surgery for medically compromised patients until such time as systemic complications are stabilised.

Those patients with relative contraindications require careful consideration. These include medical, social and compliance-related factors.

In the United Kingdom, management of patients who require antibiotic prophylaxis for endocarditis has been greatly simplified through the introduction of new guidelines from the British Society of Antimicrobial Chemotherapy (BSAC) (Gould et al., 2006). These guidelines have not, however, been universally accepted at the time of this book going to press.

Patient groups requiring antibiotic prophylaxis have been reduced to three:
• those with previous endocarditis
• those with heart valve replacement
• those with surgically constructed systemic or pulmonary shunts.

All dentogingival manipulations for these patients require antibiotic cover. There is no longer a need to provide intravenous antibiotic cover; oral antibiotic cover is now considered sufficient. Older BSAC guidelines are still published in the British National Formulary (BNF), and medicolegally either is acceptable as the guidance and advice of a recognised and properly constituted expert group.

Other relative medical contraindications should be considered practically on a case-by-case basis and treatment provided following careful appraisal of risks and assessment of response to previous surgical intervention.

Addiction poses particular problems in the management of surgical patients. Smoking is a significant risk factor for periodontal surgical failure and failure of implant placement. Alcohol dependence will predispose to excess bleeding where liver function has been impaired. It is important to consider that patients with liver disease may be thrombocytopenic as well as having abnormal clotting factor levels. In such cases, a full blood count must be taken in addition to an INR (prothrombin time). Platelet levels below 60,000/ml of whole blood represent a risk for surgical intervention. The disordered lifestyle led by some alcoholics may compromise the delivery of the planned regular care necessary for surgical success. It may be sensible to suggest other treatment approaches for these patients.

Phobic patients or those with poor compliance are generally less suitable for periodontal surgery than others. Often these procedures may be relatively time-consuming and technically demanding for the operator. Whilst conscious sedation techniques may render treatment possible for these patients, anxiety and poor coping skills may render the post-surgical phase relatively stormy and future management more difficult. Again, simpler, non-surgical treatment options may be more appropriate for such patients.

Preoperative Management

Careful preoperative management and planning will often simplify surgery itself and allow a more predictable post-operative healing phase. Meticulous record-keeping and the use of evidence-based practice should be observed in this regard.

Record-Keeping

As discussed previously, the informed consent process is vital and should be well documented. General risks are involved in any surgical procedure and should be discussed with the patient. These include pain, swelling, bruising and bleeding. Many of these can be minimised with careful technique. Risks specific to the particular procedure should also be discussed. These include, for example, gingival recession in areas of aesthetic importance and the potential for paraesthesia where surgery is in close proximity to neurovascular bundles. Consent forms are a useful adjunct in the consent process where sedation or general anaesthesia is contemplated. A copy should be retained in the patient notes and another given to the patient.

Where aesthetic change is planned or is a risk, it is valuable to obtain photographic records so that before and after comparisons may be made. Study models are also helpful in this regard. Recession defects, for example, may be monitored over time and assessed for change after surgery. Where there is chronic periodontitis, as a minimum standard an up-to-date detailed pocket chart should be recorded before any surgery is planned. Good quality contemporary radiographs are an invaluable patient record, as well as a useful aid for diagnosis and surgical planning.

Antimicrobial Chemotherapy

Periodontal inflammation is most frequently plaque-induced. Whilst surgical insult to oral mucosal tissues will also induce an inflammatory response, this will be amplified by poor preoperative plaque control and prolonged by inadequate post-operative cleaning. Prolonged inflammation will potentiate post-operative discomfort and compromise healing by primary intention.

It is important to ensure that oral hygiene is optimal prior to surgery. A 0.2% chlorhexidine gluconate mouthwash (Fig 1-1) four times daily (q.d.s.) one

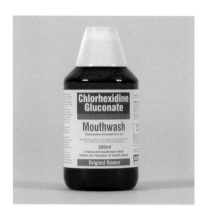

Fig 1-1 Generic chlorhexidine gluconate 0.2% mouthwash. The use of generic products, where possible, is most cost-effective.

week prior to and two weeks post-surgery is invaluable in this respect. This has been shown to reduce discomfort and promote healing (Newman and Addy, 1982). In addition, chlorhexidine used immediately preoperatively has been shown to reduce the bacterial load and aerosol contamination of the operative area and surrounding environment.

Analgesia
The notion of pre-emptive analgesia is growing in importance in surgical management. This is based on the principle that preoperative administration of NSAIDs (non-steroidal anti-inflammatory drugs) will diminish the tissue response to the cascade of pain messengers induced by surgical insult. This in turn will reduce the potential for peripheral or central sensitisation to pain and prolonged post-operative discomfort. The beneficial use of preoperative NSAIDs has been demonstrated in a number of studies. The authors would recommend a single dose of 800 mg ibuprofen preoperatively where appropriate. Currently, this drug and dosage taken three times daily represent the gold standard for pain relief. British National Formulary (BNF) guidelines would suggest commencing on 400 mg ibuprofen three times daily (t.d.s.), and this is a departure from the guidance. Practitioners should therefore exercise caution in this respect. Where ibuprofen is contraindicated owing to gastrointestinal erosion or asthma, 1000 mg of paracetamol is usually a safe alternative.

Surgical Analgesia and Haemostasis
The term "anaesthesia" is used most often in dentistry to describe the local phenomenon of absence of painful sensation following delivery of local

anaesthetic drugs. As the effect is, in fact, a local absence of pain, and patient consciousness is not altered, the term surgical analgesia is used preferentially throughout this book.

Profound analgesia is a prerequisite for high-quality periodontal surgery, and achieving this is time well spent to overcome partial or total loss of analgesia intra-operatively. Haemostasis, however, is also of critical importance as a relatively "dry" operating site will improve visibility and thus render treatment very much more predictable. The use of local anaesthetic drugs is important for delivery of these haemostatic agents (i.e. epinephrine).

Analgesia for surgery, unfortunately, is not wholly predictable. Studies have shown, for example, that a positive lip sign after administration of inferior alveolar block is a poor indicator of analgesic success (Dreven et al., 1987). The choice of local anaesthetic agent is important. The agent articaine has enjoyed widespread popularity in general practice. Anecdotally, this agent provides profound analgesia. It has not, however, been shown to be any more effective than lidocaine with 1:100,000 epinephrine (Mikesell et al., 2005). In addition, the incidence of paraesthesia with articaine has been shown to be significantly increased, presumably as a result of the increased concentration of anaesthetic agent.

Of particular significance in surgery is the concentration of vasoconstrictor agents. The use of greater concentrations of epinephrine in local anaesthetics has been shown to effect an improvement in haemostasis. In particular the use of lidocaine with 1:50,000 epinephrine (Fig 1-2) produced more than a

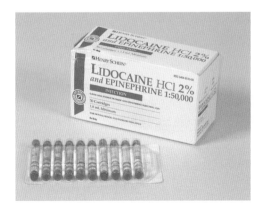

Fig 1-2 Lidocaine with 1:50,000 epinephrine.

50% improvement as compared with lidocaine with 1:100,000 epinephrine (Buckley et al., 1984). This is an effective drug for local infiltration analgesia with proven safety. The use of a slow infiltration (1 ml/minute) technique has been recommended.

Finally, in periodontal access flap or resective surgery, the use of an intrapapillary injection after sulcular or block analgesia provides additional and excellent haemostasis and a clearer visual field (Fig 1-3).

A checklist for preoperative preparation is included in Box 1-1.

Operative Management

In periodontal surgery, basic surgical principles remain the same whatever type of surgical procedure is planned. Chapter 2 will describe these basic principles. Subsequent chapters will go on to emphasise specific elements of surgical management unique to the procedure being carried out. In general terms the operative procedure should be carried out efficiently and in a timely manner.

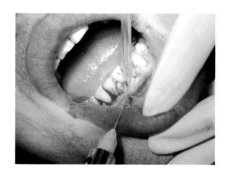

Fig 1-3 Intrapapillary injection of local anaesthetic during gingivectomy procedure. Blanching of the papilla indicates local vasoconstriction.

Box 1-1 **Preoperative checklist**

- Written consent
- Preoperative records (photos, pocket chart, study models, radiographs)
- Oral hygiene instruction and prophylaxis
- Chlorhexidine 0.2% mouthwash b.d. to begin one week prior to surgery
- Pre-emptive analgesia 800 mg ibuprofen 1 hour pre-op
  (or 1 g paracetamol)

Patient stamina will tend to reduce during a lengthy procedure. The operator must appear confident and comfortable with the procedure even where this is technically demanding. Losing patient confidence intraoperatively can make a difficult procedure even more challenging. Meticulous preparation, deliberate and careful technique, and keeping sight of specific surgical objectives will help the operator to project this confidence to their patient. It is also essential to have the skill and ability to complete a procedure quickly if a patient becomes distressed.

Post-operative Management

Achieving Post-operative Haemostasis

Haemostasis should be ensured before the patient leaves the surgery. This is usually achieved with simple pressure with a moistened gauze pad. Suturing may be suitable to control haemorrhage from the underside of a flap.

Immediate post-operative haemorrhage may be of three types:
• chronic ooze
• small vessel arterial bleed
• bone bleeding where bone-cutting has taken place.

A useful technique to manage a chronic ooze not responding to simple pressure is applying pressure with a gauze pad soaked in epinephrine containing local anaesthetic solution. If the bleed is from an open wound (e.g. gingivectomy wound), a useful tip is to mix zinc oxide powder with sterile water and with strands of cotton wool from a cotton wool roll. This is applied as a dressing to the open wound and the astringency of the zinc oxide is an excellent haemostatic agent. A protective dressing such as Coe-Pak may be placed over this (Fig 1-4).

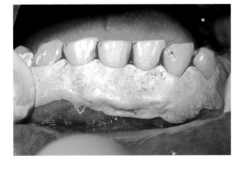

Fig 1-4 A Coe-Pak periodontal dressing after gingivectomy procedure aids haemostasis where raw tissue surfaces are exposed.

Traditional surgical dressings (e.g. Coe-Pak) were prescribed for their antimicrobial value; however, these do not, in fact, possess any substantial antimicrobial efficacy. They are helpful where interdental spaces need to be maintained patent following crown lengthening surgery or gingivectomy. They help prevent rebound tissue proliferation in the early healing phase.

Larger accessory vessels may arise from greater palatine vessels and a circumvessel suture may be needed to occlude the vessel and potentiate haemostasis. Bleeding vessels within bone (e.g. retromolar/buccal artery distal to lower molars) cannot be "tied off". In such cases it may be necessary to consider the use of a contemporary form of bone wax such as an alkylene oxide copolymer (e.g. Ostene) to occlude the bleeding vessels and gain haemostasis. These agents have the handling properties of bone wax but are biocompatible and do not create foreign body reactions.

Analgesia

Currently NSAIDs represent the gold standard for relief of dentally related pain. In particular, a regime of ibuprofen 800 mg three times daily (t.d.s.) provides the most predictable relief of discomfort. If this has not been given preoperatively it should be given immediately post-operatively. Paracetamol 1000 mg q.d.s. is an appropriate alternative where traditional NSAIDs are contraindicated. Opioid drugs may be used where pain relief is inadequate with NSAIDs. This would, however, be relatively unusual.

It is good practice to infiltrate post-surgically with a long-acting local anaesthetic such as bupivacaine 0.5% (Marcaine). This will give the patient around six to eight hours free from discomfort, which may be enough to provide a good night's sleep. A secondary effect is the prevention of central sensitisation to post-operative nociceptor activation. This has been shown to decrease post-operative use of analgesics, relative to placebo, long after the effects of anaesthesia have disappeared (Hargreaves and Keiser, 2002). Bupivacaine is available in 10 ml ampoules for hypodermic administration (Fig 1-5).

Post-operative Instructions

Where incision has involved gingival margins, tooth-brushing will be uncomfortable and potentially traumatic. The patient should be prescribed a 0.2% chlorhexidine gluconate mouthwash to use until tooth-brushing can be resumed comfortably in the surgical site. The patient should brush other sites as normal.

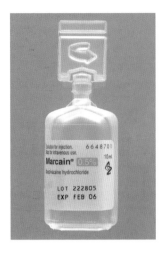

Fig 1-5 Bupivacaine 0.5% for post-operative administration. This is drawn up in a sterile syringe and injected with a hypodermic needle.

Trauma and tension to the surgical site should be discouraged and the patient should be asked to leave this alone as far as possible. This is particularly relevant to mucogingival surgery where stability of a connective tissue graft is of primary importance. A soft diet and rest are sensible after surgery. Patients should be advised to refrain from smoking and alcohol in the initial healing phase. Written post-operative instructions should be given and should include a telephone number if emergency contact is necessary.

Review Visit

It is good practice to review all surgical patients no later than one week following surgery. At this time any periodontal dressings and sutures may be removed. Where healing occurs by primary intention, sutures may be removed as early as 48 hours but by no later than four to five days. After this time sutures serve to act only as an irritant to the tissues (Selvig and Torabinejad, 1996). Sutures should be swabbed with chlorhexidine mouthwash prior to removal to avoid contaminating suture tracts with bacteria, which may result in the development of a stitch abscess (Fig 1-6).

As a general principle resorbable sutures should also be removed. Where these have been placed in deep layers, such as in connective tissue graft, or in poorly accessible areas, these may be left.

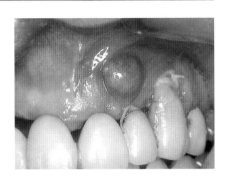

Fig 1-6 A stitch abscess has developed post-suture removal after a tissue regeneration procedure.

References

Buckley JA, Cianco SG, McMullen JA. Efficacy of epinephrine concentration in local anesthesia during periodontal surgery. J Periodontol 1984;55:653–657.

Dreven LJ, Reader A, Beck M, Meyers WJ, Weaver J. An evaluation of an electric pulp tester as a measure of analgesia in human vital teeth. J Endod 1987;13:233–238.

Gould FK, Elliott TS, Foweraker J, Fulford M, Perry JD, Roberts GJ, Sandoe JA, Watkin RW. Working Party of the British Society for Antimicrobial Chemotherapy. Guidelines for the prevention of endocarditis: report of the Working Party of the British Society for Antimicrobial Chemotherapy. J Antimicrob Chemother 2006;57:1035–1042.

Hargreaves KM, Keiser K. Development of new pain management strategies. J Dent Educ 2002;66:113–121.

Mikesell P, Nusstein J, Reader A, Beck M, Weaver J. A comparison of articaine and lidocaine for inferior alveolar nerve blocks. J Endod 2005;31:265–270.

Newman PS, Addy M. Comparison of hypertonic saline and chlorhexidine mouthrinses after the inverse bevel flap procedure. J Periodontol 1982;53:315–318.

Selvig KA, Torabinejad M. Wound healing after mucoperiosteal surgery in the cat. J Endod 1996;22:507-515.

Further Reading

Malamed SF, Gagnon S, Leblanc D. Articaine hydrochloride: a study of the safety of a new amide local anesthetic. J Am Dent Assoc 2001;132(2):177–185.

Oxford League Table of Analgesic Efficacy. www.jr2.ox.ac.uk/bandolier/ booth/painpag/Acutrev/Analgesics/lftab.html. Oxford: Bandolier, 2006.

Chapter 2
Principles and Practice of Periodontal Surgery 2: Basic Surgical Principles

Aim

The aim of this chapter is to explore the principles underpinning contemporary periodontal surgery by guiding the reader through the various stages of surgery. The text will describe modern surgical equipment and methods and contrast this with more traditional armamentaria and approaches.

Outcome

Having read this chapter, the reader will be aware of general surgical techniques applicable to all aspects of periodontal surgery. The practitioner will understand the value and use of microsurgical methods and how these principles can be transferred to their own surgical practice.

Introduction

Periodontal surgery encompasses a broad range of procedures involving the supporting tissues of the teeth. These vary in complexity from simple exodontia to technically demanding periodontal plastic surgery and include the management of periodontal and endodontic disease, preparation for and placement of implants, and preparatory treatment for fixed and removable prostheses (preprosthetic surgery).

Periodontal surgical methods were practised in Roman times when diseased gingival tissues were excised with crude instruments and without local anaesthetic. Burning of the tissue was considered an important step in the cure of disease. The last five years, however, have embraced rapid changes in therapeutic techniques owing to our greater understanding of the biological principles of healing and the consequences of surgical insult. Modern surgical management reflects both a move towards evidence-based practice and the introduction of improved techniques and instrumentation.

Whilst the complexity of microsurgery may not be routinely necessary in general dental practice, many of the principles and equipment used do improve the ease and predictability of standard surgical management.

Tenets of Halsted

Many of the principles of modern day surgery are based on the teaching of William Halsted from the late nineteenth century. He scorned common surgical practices that relied on brute strength and in their place espoused careful and gentle tissue handling. His mastectomy operation for breast cancer revolutionised what was once a uniformly fatal disease. He also introduced the use of rubber gloves to surgery.

Contemporary surgical practice recognises the "Tenets of Halsted" (Box 2-1). These tenets still stand as guiding principles in periodontal surgery.

Box 2-1 **Tenets of Halsted**

1. The gentle handling of tissues.
2. An aseptic technique.
3. Sharp anatomic dissection of tissues.
4. Careful haemostasis, using fine, non-irritating suture material in minimal amounts.
5. The obliteration of dead space in the wound.
6. The avoidance of tension.
7. The importance of rest.

Operative Management

Meticulous technique and careful tissue-handling married with microsurgical instrumentation will provide predictable and aesthetic healing in the majority of cases. Magnification using loupes is invaluable for periodontal surgery. The limited field of the operating microscope can make periodontal surgical management taxing where a broader visual field is required. Specific surgical techniques will be applicable to particular flap designs and procedures. The following form generic guiding principles for operative surgical management.

Flap Design
A myriad of flap designs exist in periodontal surgery. Commonly used flap types and their synonyms are presented in Table 2-1 (pages 15, 16 and 17).

Table 2-1 **Common flap types: advantages and disadvantages** (continued on pages 16 and 17)

Flap descriptor	Secondary descriptor	Description detail	Advantages	Disadvantages	Uses
Flap geometry	**Marginal**	Incision follows gingival margins			
	Simple replaced flap (envelope flap) Modified Widman flap	Intrasulcular incision around teeth of interest (modified Widman involves a parasulcular incision prior to the sulcular incision)	Simple, quick Replacement and suturing is simple	Access is limited to coronal aspects of root in most instances	Exodontia. Simple root surface debridement (RSD) Guided tissue regeneration (GTR)
	Two-sided flap (triangular flap)	Intrasulcular incision with one vertical relieving incision	Better access to deep periodontal lesions or root apices	Access is limited where roots are long or horizontal component of flap is short	Exodontia. Periradicular surgery RSD deep sites Root resection
	Three-sided flap	Intrasulcular incision with bilateral vertical relieving incisions	Best access of all flap types	Replacement may be demanding Where horizontal component of flap is short, blood supply may be compromised	Any periodontal surgery where maximum access is required

Table 2-1 **Common flap types: advantages and disadvantages** (continued)

Flap descriptor	Secondary descriptor	Description detail	Advantages	Disadvantages	Uses
Flap geometry	**Submarginal** Incision apical to marginal gingivae				
	Semilunar flap	Incision made over roots of interest	Quick and simple No marginal recession	Access is usually fairly limited and these flap designs are now relatively outmoded for this reason	Used for periradicular surgery
	Trapezoidal flap				
	Ochsenbein–Luebke flap				
Flap thickness	Full thickness (muco-periosteal)	Incision down to bone, flap raised from bone with blunt dissection	Good access to bone and root surface Simple procedure Minimal post-operative discomfort	Unsuitable for grafting – does not offer vascular bed Limited mobility of flap	Most periodontal surgical procedures
	Split thickness (mucosal)	Most often a three-sided design but variable Sharp dissection of tissues leaves periosteum intact	Provides good blood supply for grafts Avoids exposure dehiscence	Technically demanding Greater post-operative discomfort No access to underlying bone or root surface	Used for free gingival or connective tissue grafting

Flap descriptor	Secondary descriptor	Description detail	Advantages	Disadvantages	Uses
Replacement position	Replaced flap	Flap margins are replaced in original position	Best closure and haemostasis Healing by primary intention	Not suitable for grafting or some crown-lengthening procedures	Used for most periodontal surgery
	Repositioned flap (coronally, apically, laterally)	Margins replaced in altered relationship	Allows coverage of defects, grafts or exposure of tooth substance	Healing by secondary intention Technically demanding	Used for mucogingival surgery and crown lengthening

In general most flaps can be described as having a horizontal and a vertical component. The horizontal component of the flap normally involves an intrasulcular or parasulcular incision around the gingival margins of the teeth of interest. The vertical component of the flap is also known as a relieving incision. This helps to relieve tissue tension and allow greater access to the periradicular tissues. Ideally a flap should solely involve an intrasulcular incision for surgical access (envelope flap). This design is also referred to as a simple replaced flap and is utilised for open root surface debridement or where simple access for surgical exodontia is required. Where there is a need for greater access or relief of tissue tension, vertical relieving incisions may be employed. In general, two relieving incisions (a three-sided flap) provide optimal access to the surgical site and reduce tissue tension (Fig 2-1).

One relieving incision (a two-sided flap), however, may provide adequate access and improved blood supply and may reduce the number of sutures required for closure (Fig 2-2).

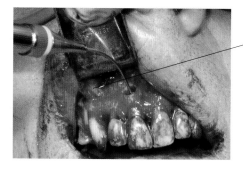

Circumoral muscular attachment

Fig 2-1 A large three-sided flap provides excellent access for root-end filling during periradicular surgery. Muscle attachment is visible on the right-hand side.

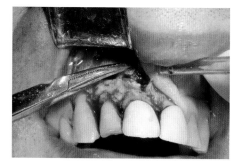

Fig 2-2 A two-sided flap with a wide horizontal component can provide excellent access.

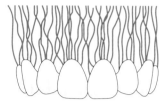

Fig 2-3a Schematic diagram of gingival blood vessels.

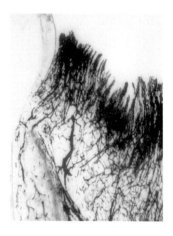

Fig 2-3b A photomicrograph of a histological section from a dog demonstrates the orientation of gingival vasculature (stained in black).

Animal research has demonstrated that gingival blood vessels tend to have a relatively vertical orientation (Fig 2-3a,b). Incisions, therefore, should be as vertically orientated as possible to minimise bisecting these vessels. This approach will reduce intra-operative bleeding and also maximise blood supply to the tissues surrounding the raised flap. Maintaining a flap base at least as broad as the coronal incision will ensure an adequate blood supply. Where there is a relatively oblique incision, however, this may compromise the blood supply to the bound tissue beneath the flap. In general, the significant collateral circulation present within the gingival tissues obviates any risks of ischaemic flap necrosis secondary to a compromised blood supply. Flap perfusion has been shown to be compromised where the ratio of flap length to width is greater than 2:1 (Patterson, 1968). Where this is a potential risk, the operator should extend flap width horizontally.

A flap may also be described as full or partial (split) thickness:

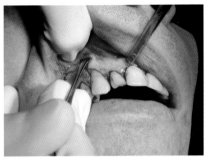

Fig 2-4 Raising a full-thickness flap.

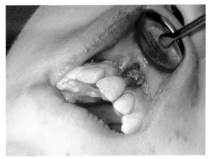

Fig 2-5 A partial-thickness flap.

- A full thickness flap involves complete incision through the gingival tissues down to bone. When the flap is raised the periosteal layer is stripped from the surface of the alveolar bone using the bone as a fulcrum point (Fig 2-4). This flap is the most frequently used in periodontal access surgery.
- The partial thickness flap (Fig 2-5) is created by incision through gingival tissues but stopping short of contact with bone. A sharp dissection technique is used subsequently when raising the mucosal flap in order to separate the mucosa from the periosteum, which is left *in situ* adapted to the underlying bone. This flap is most commonly used for mucogingival grafting or pedicle–flap transfer procedures.

A useful contemporary technique in periodontal surgery involves papilla-preservation flaps (Fig 2-6). These may be particularly useful in implant surgery or periapical root surgery. One variation described by Velvart

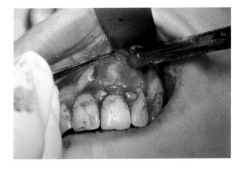

Fig 2-6 A papilla-sparing flap. When the flap is raised, papillae are left *in situ*.

(Velvart, 2002) describes an intrasulcular incision around the cervical margin and the preparation of a split-thickness flap at the base of the interdental papillae. Where papillae have not been raised, the potential for papillary recession and subsequent unaesthetic "black triangles" is greatly reduced.

Incision

Sharp anatomic dissection forms one of the important tenets of Halsted critical to modern surgical management. Microsurgical instruments and techniques have made this goal achievable in the technically demanding region of the gingival margin. The Swann-Morton fine range includes microsurgical blades contoured to allow accurate dissection around gingival margins (Fig 2-7). Round, textured handles permit fine manual control of the microsurgical blades (Fig 2-8). They are not prohibitively expensive and represent a simple change that will improve surgical management of the gingival margin immensely.

The traditional blade shapes still retain an important place in surgical management. In particular, the number 15 blade is designed to allow good contact with bone and is invaluable for vertical relieving incisions (Fig 2-9).

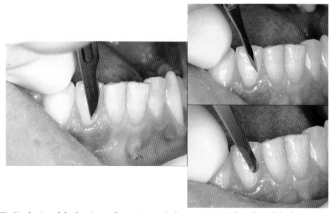

Fig 2-7 Relative blade sizes for gingival dissection. The first blade is a standard size 15. This can be contrasted with SP90 (spear shape) and SM64 microblades.

Fig 2-8 Micro-
surgical blade and
handle.

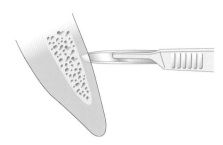

Fig 2-9 Curved end of 15 blade cutting onto bone.

Where the vertical relieving incision meets the gingival margin, a 90° angle should be made by changing blade inclination (Fig 2-10). Acute margins are more difficult to close and are also prone to local ischaemic necrosis.

The number 12 blade design may be useful for posterior intrasulcular incisions (Fig 2-11). Angled handles also permit improved access for posterior regions or gingivectomy procedures (Fig 2-12).

Blake knives (Fig 2-13) represent a useful addition for periodontal surgery, particularly gingivectomy procedures. Here the blade is at an acute angle to the instrument handle. These instruments are, however, relatively difficult to assemble and clean, and leave the operator and assistant more prone to sharps injury.

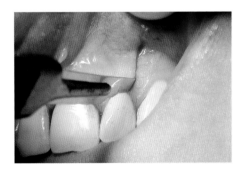

Fig 2-10 Terminating vertical relieving incision at 90° to the gingival margin.

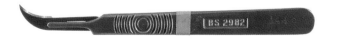

Fig 2-11
No. 12 blade.

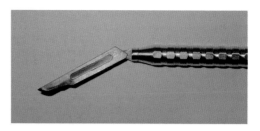

Fig 2-12 Angled handle.

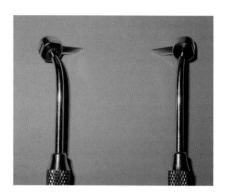

Fig 2-13 Blake knives.

Finally, it is recommended that incisions are made at least twice to ensure periosteal breach and facilitate gentle flap reflection/elevation. Often a mucoperiosteal flap will start to elevate with the second incision.

Reflection
Traditionally, the Howarth's pattern elevator (also called nasal rasparatory) has been used for tissue elevation (Fig 2-14). This particular elevator is, however, relatively blunt. The use of blunt or misdirected elevators may

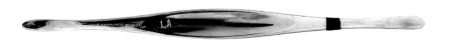

Fig 2-14 Howarth's nasal rasparatory.

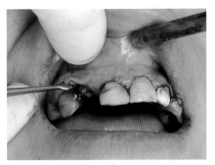

Fig 2-15 Papillary elevation.

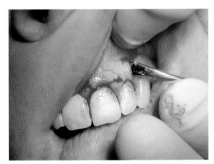

Fig 2-16 Sharp-edged elevator (Hu–Friedy 24G).

incur damage to the flap and impair subsequent healing. They may render flap elevation more difficult and time-consuming as they are difficult to introduce into the subperiosteal tissue plane. Modern periodontal surgery relies on sharp elevators to efficiently cleave periosteum from bone. Examples include the Buser papilla elevator, which includes a fine spear-shaped portion for papillary elevation (Fig 2-15), and the Hu–Friedy 24G elevator, which has a sharp, curved portion to lift the remaining flap (Fig 2-16). The use of a flat plastic instrument may also be valuable for papillary elevation. Its small size helps to minimise crush trauma to these delicate tissues.

The corner of horizontal and vertical relieving incisions is often the easiest place to begin raising a flap as tissue tension here is low. It is often possible to undermine the flap with a horizontal approach through the vertical relieving incision. If gingival margins have been carefully dissected these should lift easily from the marginal bone. Where difficulty in lifting papillae is experienced, the operator should retrace the original intrasulcular incision for a third time if necessary.

Retraction
Numerous patterns of retractors are available. Adequate retraction of the flap will allow good vision of the surgical field of interest and help to hold the lips and buccal tissues out of the way (Fig 2-17). Useful retractors include the Minnesota, Carr and Kim–Percora retractors; the retractor choice is very much down to operator preference.

Flap retraction should also allow room for instruments specific to the operative procedure. It is important not to impinge on flap tissue with

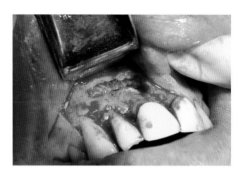

Fig 2-17 Minnesota retractor.

retractors as this will cause localised ischaemia and potentially induce bruising, which may result in impaired healing. Retractors may also be useful for tissue protection particularly on the lingual aspect of mandibular third molars. Damage to retractors with rotary instruments should be avoided where possible; this may shorten the lifespan of instruments and potentially leave metal fragments in the surgical site. The use of elevators as retractors is discouraged. Again, damage to these instruments (Fig 2-16) will impair their efficiency and reduce their lifespan. Damaged instruments are also harder to clean and autoclave.

Bone Management

In many instances bone removal (ostectomy) is important to the success of a procedure. Examples include crown-lengthening surgery, periradicular surgery and third molar exodontia. Bone removal may involve the use of either hand or rotary instruments. The mainstay of ostectomy management under local analgaesia is rotary instrumentation.

Bone has been shown to be particularly sensitive to changes in temperature (Eriksson and Albrektsson, 1984), with an increase of 10°C for one minute sufficient to induce necrosis and impaired regeneration. Whilst this is particularly relevant for implant surgery, operators should take care to avoid excessive heating of bone for any periodontal surgery. Rotary instruments should therefore be used with minimal pressure and intermittent cutting strokes. Cutting speed has been shown to be relevant in this regard, with high-speed cutting associated with less temperature increase than low speed (Agren and Arwill, 1968). The main risk of surgical emphysema from high-speed turbine handpieces has been overcome by modern, back-venting

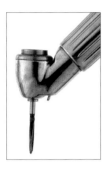

Fig 2-18 Lindemann bone burr in Impact Air 45° handpiece.

surgical turbines. An example includes the Impact Air 45° (Fig 2-18). This has been designed with a 45° head angle to improve access for resection of roots of third molar teeth. It is also very useful for apical root-end resection. Tactile feedback is very different with this instrument relative to the traditional slow-speed handpiece, and care should therefore be taken not to overcut. The use of coolant is mandatory and this should be accurately directed to the cutting edge of the burr.

Burr choice plays an important role in ostectomy. Diamond burrs have been shown to clog with bone particles and increase frictional heat (Moss, 1964) and are therefore not recommended. The use of round or fissure burrs with widely spaced flutes, such as the Lindemann bone-cutting burr, are useful alternatives (Fig 2-18).

Fine removal of bone is sometimes required in crown-lengthening surgery where all attempts are made to avoid damage to adjacent root structure. Initially, rotary instruments should be used to leave a thin layer of bone overlying root structure. The subsequent use of hand instruments such as fine chisels or sharp curettes will then permit safe removal of the thin plate of residual bone, avoiding root surface damage.

Flap Compression and Closure
Careful apposition of wound margins is essential to aid uneventful healing by primary intention and to maintain optimal soft tissue aesthetics. The surgical site should be debrided with sterile saline prior to definitive closure. It is helpful to position the flap in an ideal position prior to closure. This is particularly useful where changes in flap position are planned, for example an apically-repositioned flap.

It is good practice to compress a flap with moistened gauze after closure and suturing for about one minute, and also to do this prior to suturing to minimise dead tissue space and potential haematoma formation.

Suture choice plays an important role. The use of black silk in oral surgery is now regarded as outmoded. This material readily wicks (soaks up) tissue fluids and is rapidly colonised with bacteria (Fig 2-19). Synthetic monofilament materials have grown in popularity in periodontal surgery. These materials do not wick tissue fluids and exhibit minimal bacterial colonisation (Fig 2-20). They do not, however, tie as well as silk, and knots may loosen over time. A useful tip is to "lock" the suture after the tie is made. This is achieved with a firm tugging pressure in the opposite direction to that with which the suture has been tied (Fig 2-21). Cut ends of sutures may be sharp and relatively irritating to the patient. Braided coated synthetic materials represent a marriage of the handling properties of silk and the biological compatibility of the synthetic materials. Resorbable materials are useful where buried sutures have to be placed, for example connective tissue grafting, or where removal may be technically demanding or uncomfortable for the patient. As a principle, these sutures should not be left in the oral environment as they will be readily colonised by bacteria.

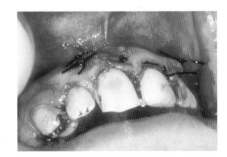

Fig 2-19 Poor healing response to black silk sutures.

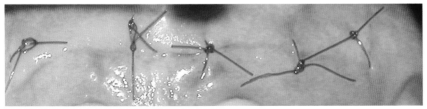

Fig 2-20 Healing response with 5.0 Prolene.

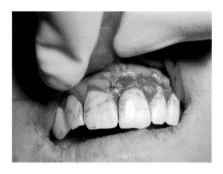

Fig 2-21 Tight tying pressure on suture at 90° to the original direction of tie will lock the suture knot in place.

Cutting-type needles will make flap penetration easier but increase flap damage and the risk of "pull through". Reverse-cutting needles will decrease the risk of suture "pull-through". Non-cutting needles are more resistant to tissue passage but may be more suitable for very delicate tissues, such as connective tissue graft or lingual mucosa.

Selection of suture size is important. For closure of bleeding sockets or where healing by secondary intention is expected, 3-0 and 4-0 sutures are most suitable. Meticulous flap closure, however, relies on smaller diameter sutures, from 5-0 to 8-0. It is more difficult to close flaps under tension with fine diameter materials as they will tend to snap. This is advantageous, as flap closure under tension will lead to bunching of tissues and ischaemic regions, and impaired healing, potentially with scar formation. It is more difficult to see small diameter suture materials. Magnification is useful for 5-0 sutures and mandatory for sutures finer than this.

Needle length and shape are important in different areas. For fine aesthetic anterior work, a short needle of 5 mm greatly simplifies tissue manipulation. Short needles will not pass through wide interdental embrasures, and 15 mm is probably a more appropriate length where posterior teeth are involved.

A good-quality suturing kit represents an important investment for a periodontal surgeon (Fig 2-22). This should include fine needle holders, tissue pickups and sharp scissors.

There are several different methods for suturing in the oral cavity, and to describe each method is beyond the scope of this chapter. The most commonly used and versatile technique for suturing in dentistry is the simple interrupted suture (Chapter 4). Sutures should be tightened sufficiently to

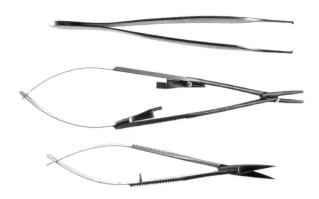

Fig 2-22 Micro-
surgical suture kit.

approximate the edges of the flap without undue tension. In general, needle penetration should be placed so that the wound edges meet at the same level. This will minimise the possibility of mismatched wound edge heights. The "bite" of the needle in soft tissue should allow at least 2 mm from the edge of the flap to prevent the suture tearing through the mucosa.

The application of a periodontal dressing is useful when bone or raw tissue surfaces are left exposed. This may improve patient comfort and also prevent trauma or contamination of the surgical site.

Box 2-2 describes a simple microsurgical kit suitable for most periodontal surgical procedures. It is impractical to be prescriptive in this respect as practitioners will find that certain instruments work better in their own hands. These suggestions are only those that work well for the authors.

Box 2-2 **Basic microsurgical kit**

- Microsurgical blade handle (Swann Morton fine range)
- Sharp, fine elevator (Buser papilla elevator)
- Fine tissue pickups (Micro Adson forceps)
- Fine needle holders (Castroviejo pattern)
- Fine scissors (Castroviejo pattern)

Disposables
- Microblades (Swann Morton SM64)
- Fine sutures (6-0 Prolene, Ethicon)

The introduction of modern techniques and an evidence base to periodontal surgery has helped to simplify management and allow for comfortable aesthetic healing in the majority of cases. Simple changes to technique can be inexpensive and will let the surgeon and the patient enjoy a more pleasant and predictable operative experience.

References

Agren E, Arwill T. High-speed or conventional dental equipment for the removal of bone in oral surgery. 3. A histologic and microradiographic study on bone repair in the rabbit. Acta Odontol Scand 1968;26:223–246.

Eriksson RA, Albrektsson T. The effect of heat on bone regeneration: an experimental study in the rabbit using the bone growth chamber. J Oral Maxillofac Surg 1984;42:705–711.

Moss RW. Histopathologic reaction of bone to surgical cutting. Oral Surg Oral Med Oral Pathol 1964;405–414.

Patterson TJ. The survival of skin flaps in the pig. Br J Plast Surg 1968;21:113–117.

Velvart P. Papilla base incision: a new approach to recession-free healing of the interdental papilla after endodontic surgery. Int Endod J 2002;35:453–460.

Further Reading

Silverstein LH. Principles of Dental Suturing: The complete guide to surgical closure. New Jersey: Montage Media Corp, 2000:8–77.

Chapter 3

Surgical Management of Gingival Overgrowth

Aim

To provide a brief overview of the aetiology of gingival overgrowth, and describe the principles of and techniques for its surgical management.

Outcome

Having read this chapter, the reader should be aware of the contemporary surgical techniques used for the surgical management of gingival overgrowth. It is hoped that the reader will understand which types of gingival enlargement are amenable to surgical treatment and be aware of alternative key management strategies. The principal causes and non-surgical management of gingival overgrowth have been discussed in detail in Chapters 5 and 6 of book 43/44 in this series (*Periodontal Medicine – A Window on the Body*) and are beyond the scope of this chapter.

Introduction

Gingival overgrowth, gingival hyperplasia, gingival enlargement and gingival hypertrophy are terms that are used interchangeably (and incorrectly) in the literature. The term gingival overgrowth will be used for the remainder of this chapter.

Gingival overgrowth has numerous causes. These include:
• plaque-induced inflammatory swelling
• drug therapy
• systemic illness
• genetic disorders
• other specific physiologic states.

Inflammatory changes within the gingival tissues may cause enlargement of the gingivae without apical migration of the junctional epithelial attachment. Probing depths increase as a consequence and a "false pocket" is formed. Local plaque accumulation may, in fact, allow progression to chronic periodontitis and formation of true pocketing if left untreated.

Box 3-1 lists types of gingival overgrowth that may require surgical management.

Box 3-1 **Types of gingival overgrowth that may require surgical management**

Hereditary gingival fibromatosis
Drug-induced gingival overgrowth

Inflammatory gingival overgrowth due to plaque accumulation secondary to:
• orthodontic appliances
• dentures
• mouth breathing
• incompetent lip seal
• dental crowding

Gingival epulides
• fibrous epulis
• vascular epulis
• giant cell epulis

Drug-induced Gingival Overgrowth
Gingival overgrowth is a well-documented and unwanted side effect, associated principally with the calcium channel blockers, phenytoin and ciclosporin (Table 3-1). The tissue enlargement begins as a painless, bead-like enlargement of the interdental papilla and can extend to involve the buccal and lingual gingival margins. The enlargement is usually generalised but the maxillary and mandibular anterior teeth are frequently the most severely affected.

Drug-induced gingival overgrowth has two components:
1. A fibrous component which is caused by the drug (Fig 3-1).
2. An inflammatory component which is induced by plaque (Fig 3-2).

Treatment of drug-induced overgrowth and prevention of recurrence can be challenging, and the primary course of action is to attempt to remove the causative agent (drug) from the patient's medical regime. Medical management by drug substitution is, however, not always possible in patients with severe and poorly controlled epilepsy or hypertension.

Table 3-1 **Drugs that can contribute to drug-induced gingival overgrowth**

Drug Type	Uses
Calcium channel blockers	1. Hypertension. 2. Reduction of nephrotoxic effects of ciclosporin in organ transplant patients.
Phenytoin	1. Anticonvulsant. 2. Occasionally used to manage trigeminal neuralgia.
Ciclosporin	1. Potent immunosuppressant used to prevent rejection after organ or tissue transplantation. 2. Management of severe autoimmune disease, e.g. rheumatoid arthritis, ulcerative colitis, which do not respond to conventional therapy.

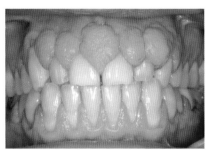

Fig 3-1 Fibrous overgrowth in a patient medicated with ciclosporin.

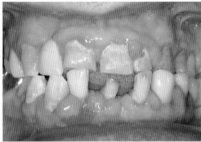

Fig 3-2 Drug-induced gingival overgrowth in a patient medicated with nifedipine. Tissues appear more vascular because of poor plaque control.

Inflammatory Gingival Overgrowth

Provision of an orthodontic appliance, especially a fixed appliance, often has a tendency to favour the accumulation of plaque around the gingival margins. This inflammation is usually transient and does not lead to attachment loss. As a result, hyperplastic tissue can lead to false pocketing around brackets and bands. This usually resolves following debonding and improvement in plaque control; surgical intervention is rarely necessary.

Low-grade, chronic irritation from an ill-fitting denture may result in an inflammatory fibrous overgrowth at the denture border. Treatment involves relieving over-extended areas of the denture. If the enlargement does not resolve, simple surgical excision is often required with subsequent provision of a new denture.

Gingival overgrowth is often seen in patients who mouth-breathe. In mouth-breathers there is increased lip separation and decreased coverage of the teeth by the upper lip (Fig 3-3). Thus there may be a decrease in saliva, which reduces the natural cleansing (plaque removal) processes. This, in turn, may contribute to increased plaque levels and subsequent gingival inflammation.

In a crowded dentition plaque control can be more difficult, leading to plaque retention and gingival overgrowth (Fig 3-4).

Epulides

Epulides are benign localised enlargements of the gingival tissues that usually develop following irritation by subgingival plaque, retained by calculus or ledges on restorations. The true epulides include:

- pyogenic granuloma (pregnancy epulis) (Fig 3-5)
- fibrous epulis (fibroepithelial polyp)
- giant cell epulis.

The aetiology and non-surgical management of epulides are covered in book 43/44 in this series and are beyond the scope of this chapter. Surgical excision

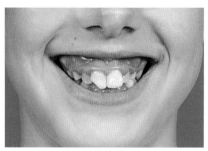

Fig 3-3 A mouth breather. Note the gingival overgrowth and high lip line.

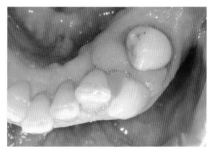

Fig 3-4 Dental crowding with gingival overgrowth. This has resulted in distal movement of the left mandibular first pre-molar.

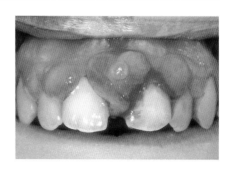

Fig 3-5 Pregnancy epulis. The tissue is highly vascular and bleeds readily.

is by gingivectomy. Prior to excision biopsy it is important to determine whether the lesion base is sessile (broad-based) or pedunculated (narrow stem). A pedunculated lesion is more straightforward to excise but more likely to have a vascular supply, and therefore it may be more haemorrhagic. Preoperative radiographs are also essential to exclude the risk of intraosseous involvement (see later).

Hereditary Gingival Fibromatosis

Hereditary gingival fibromatosis (HGF) is a rare, benign familial condition. It is characterised by proliferative, fibrous overgrown gingivae, usually of a normal colour, firm consistency and with abundant stippling. It typically develops as an isolated disorder but can be a feature of other syndromes and is inherited as an autosomal dominant or recessive condition.

The severity of HGF varies between patients and ranges from minor localised gingival enlargement to involvement of buccal and lingual attached gingival tissues in both the mandible and the maxilla. It typically affects the maxillary tuberosity (Fig 3-6) and mandibular retromolar regions (Fig 3-7).

There is no curative treatment for HGF; tissues can be debulked surgically with varying degrees of success. When the enlargement is minimal, scaling of teeth and meticulous oral hygiene may be all that is required to maintain relative stability. As the enlarged tissue increases, false pocketing develops and this, alongside aesthetic and functional problems, may necessitate surgical intervention to restore optimal gingival contours.

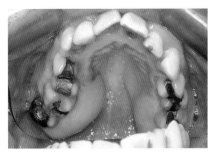

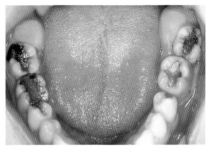

Fig 3-6 Hereditary gingival fibromatosis affecting the maxillary tuberosities.

Fig 3-7 Hereditary gingival fibromatosis affecting the mandibular retromolar regions.

Presurgical Management

Non-surgical management of gingival overgrowth should always be the first approach. This reduces the extent of plaque-induced gingival inflammation, producing a less vascular tissue bed upon which to operate. Subsequent surgical intervention becomes more straightforward and the risks of recurrence reduce. In some cases where the inflammatory component to the enlargement is substantial, a non-surgical approach may reduce the overgrowth to acceptable levels and thus avoid the need for surgery.

Non-surgical management should involve:
- A meticulous oral hygiene regime.
- Frequent professional removal of supra- and subgingival plaque and calculus, with the use of local anaesthetic if necessary.
- For drug-induced gingival overgrowth, joint management with the patient's medical specialist may be necessary to consider substitution of existing medication. Alternative medication should be considered for all patients, in line with the philosophy that medical problems should be managed medically rather than surgically. If a drug substitution is made, it is essential to allow several months after discontinuation of the original drug for resolution of the gingival overgrowth prior to a decision to intervene surgically.

Reasons for Surgical Intervention
When non-surgical therapy fails to resolve the overgrowth to a satisfactory level, surgical intervention often provides a good short-term outcome.

Indeed, surgery may establish a dentogingival complex that is more conducive to home care, thereby providing medium-term stability.

Surgical management may be indicated in the following situations:
• Plaque control is hindered or difficult.
• There is reduced masticatory efficiency due to enlarged tissues.
• Aesthetic problems. Many patients are self-conscious about the appearance of enlarged gingivae and find severe overgrowth disfiguring.
• Failure of tooth eruption. In severe cases, the gingivae can be so grossly enlarged that the teeth become buried or fail to erupt.
• Movement of teeth. Severely fibrosed tissue may lead to tooth migration; this can also lead to discomfort.
• There is interference with speech.
• There is trauma from occlusal contact with overgrown tissues.
• A biopsy is required for definitive diagnosis, where a clinical diagnosis is proving difficult.

Some Medical Considerations

Some patients may require antibiotic prophylaxis prior to procedures involving dento-gingival manipulation. These include patients with previous infective endocarditis, cardiac valve replacement surgery, or surgically constructed systemic or pulmonary shunts or conduits. The current British Society for Antimicrobial Chemotherapy (BSAC) guidelines do not recommend antibiotic prophylaxis for individuals with renal disease who require dental procedures that are likely to give rise to a bacteraemia. There are occasions, however, where antibiotic prophylaxis may be important for renal patients. Specifically, patients who are in, or have undergone, chronic renal failure will have experienced chronic hypercalcaemia, and a cardiovascular assessment is necessary to ascertain whether they have developed cardiac valve calcification secondary to this. If there is any doubt, it is necessary to contact the patient's nephrologist for clarification prior to elective dental treatment. For some patients, for example those taking systemic steroids, it is advisable to monitor their blood pressure prior to and throughout surgery.

Surgical Management

Gingivectomy

Gingivectomy literally means "excision of gingival tissue", but frequently involves the elimination of false pocketing by resection of gingival tissue. *Gingivoplasty* is the surgical recontouring of the surface of the gingiva without reducing its marginal-apical height. This is normally performed to produce a more favourable dento-gingival contour to aid oral hygiene. When there is enlargement of the gingivae, these two procedures are usually performed simultaneously. Conventional periodontal surgical principles apply, and these have been outlined in Chapters 1 and 2.

If the aetiology of the lesion is unknown or unconfirmed, a tissue sample should be sent for histopathological examination.

The aims of the gingivectomy procedure are to:
• eliminate false pocketing
• achieve an optimum gingival contour
• reduce fibrous enlargement for functional or aesthetic reasons.

It is very important to assess the amount of keratinised tissue present at the planning stage. Ideally, at least 3 mm of keratinised tissue in the apicocoronal direction should remain following excision (Fig 3-8a). If the initial gingivectomy incision is close to or at the mucogingival junction, a gingivectomy procedure should be avoided as this may eliminate keratinised tissue and predispose to problems such as recession in susceptible patients.

Analgesia is administered by regional and direct infiltration of an epinephrine-containing local anaesthetic into the enlarged tissue including individual interdental papillae (Fig 3-8b). This will improve haemostatic control intraoperatively and provide a clearer visual field for surgical re-contouring.

The deepest point of each pocket is measured with a graduated probe (Fig 3-8c) and marked on the outer gingivae by horizontal probing to create a

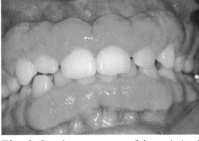

Fig 3-8a Assessment of keratinised tissue, preoperative photograph.

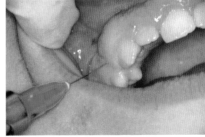

Fig 3-8b Placement of local anaesthetic solution directly into the papilla, following initial sulcular infiltrations.

bleeding point (Fig 3-8d). This resulting series of bleeding points can be used as a guideline for the initial scalloped external bevel incision. This external bevel incision is made with either a Blake knife (Fig 3-8e) or a knife with a 45° angled handle (Fig 2-12) and number 15 blade. The blade should be inclined at 45° to the long axis of the roots and the incision kept apical to the bleeding points (Fig 3-8f).

An intrasulcular incision is then made with a number 15 scalpel or with a microsurgical blade (Fig 3-8g). This releases the junctional epithelium and linked tissue, which can then be removed with a curette (Fig 3-8h). Any remaining tissue tags can also be removed using a sharp curette. Gingivoplasty is then performed with sharp blades to smooth the incision edges and to restore a healthy and aesthetic physiological contour (Fig 3-8i). Scaling and root surface debridement should be carried out at this stage.

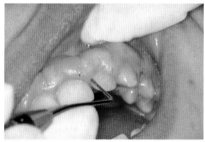

Fig 3-8c The deepest point of each pocket is measured with a graduated probe.

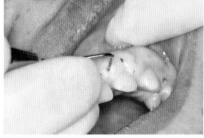

Fig 3-8d The deepest point is marked on the outer gingivae using a probe to produce a bleeding point.

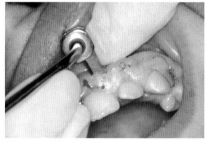

Fig 3-8e External bevel incision is made with a Blake knife.

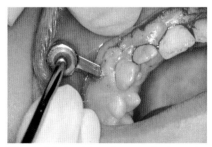

Fig 3-8f Incision kept apical to the bleeding points.

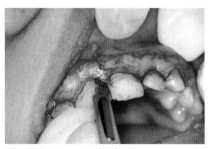

Fig 3-8g Intrasulcular incision made with a number 15 blade.

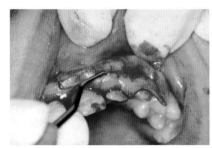

Fig 3-8h Tissue removal using a curette.

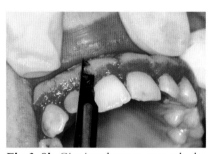

Fig 3-8i Gingivoplasty to smooth the incision edges.

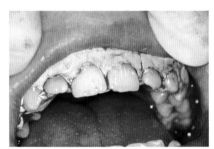

Fig 3-8j Periodontal dressing (Coe-Pak)

Electrosurgery and laser therapy may be useful alternative treatments or adjuncts to conventional surgical gingivectomy techniques, but they are less forgiving and post-operative tissue contours are less predictable.

The gingivectomy procedure leaves exposed gingival tissue and therefore relies upon healing by secondary intention. This may cause discomfort and occasionally an increased risk of post-operative haemorrhage. In these instances it is advisable to apply a periodontal dressing (Fig 3-8j), the method for which is outlined later in this chapter.

Potential adverse events from gingivectomy procedures include:
- post-operative pain/discomfort
- healing by secondary intention, which may be slow
- risk of bone exposure
- excessive removal of attached gingivae
- tooth sensitivity following exposure of root dentine, where an underlying periodontitis coexists.

Inverse Bevel Incisions for Tissue Debulking

An inverse bevel incision, parallel to the gingival sulcus, can also be used to treat gingival overgrowth when the alveolar bone needs to be accessed for osseous recontouring purposes or in areas with limited keratinised tissue. It is also used in cases of severe enlargement involving both the keratinised attached gingivae and extending apically beyond the mucogingival junction (Fig 3-9a). Debulking may necessitate flap elevation and thinning by sharp dissection from the underside of the flap (normally a split-thickness flap). In this way, keratinised tissue is preserved and primary wound closure is achieved, providing less post-operative discomfort and improved tissue contours. The sequence in Fig 3-9a–f is a schematic representation of this technique and Fig 3-10a–g illustrates a clinical case.

Fig 3-9 Diagram to illustrate the inverse bevel incision prior to flap reflection and "filleting" of the bulk of the sub-mucosal connective tissue.

(a) Bulky tissue prior to split-thickness flap reflection.

(b) First incision is parallel to a sulcus incision, using an inverse bevel.

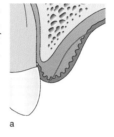
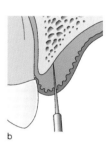

(c) Second incision isolates a tissue "cuff".

(d) Flap is then raised by sharp dissection allowing surgical access to the underside of the flap.

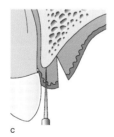
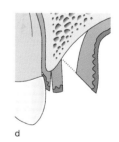

(e) Cuff is removed and underside of flap is debulked by sharp excision of excess connective tissue. Care must be taken to avoid puncturing the flap.

(f) Flap is closed after any necessary debridement and removal of the bulky connective tissue from the underside of the flap.

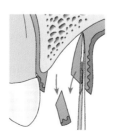
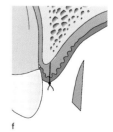

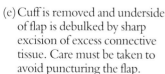

41

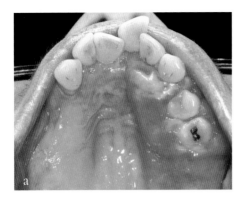

Fig 3-10a Grossly expanded gingival tissues extending apical to mucogingival junction. Conventional open-face gingivectomy was not a surgical option in this case.

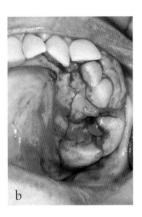

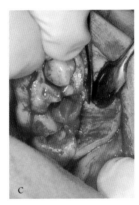

Fig 3-10b (left) Inverse bevel incisions parallel to the sulcus and following extraction of maxillary left 4 and 5.

Fig 3-10c (right) Elevation of buccal flap leaving buccal tissue wedge to excise.

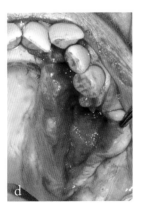

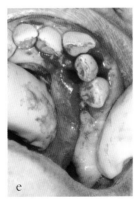

Fig 3-10d (left) Buccal and palatal flaps elevated following removal of buccal and palatal tissue wedges for initial debulking.

Fig 3-10e (right) Initial approximation of flap margins to gauge the degree of filleting required from the underside of the flaps to achieve optimal post-operative tissue contours.

Fig 3-10f (left) Further undermining of the palatal flap by sharp dissection.

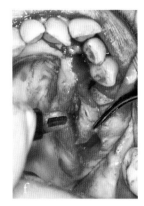 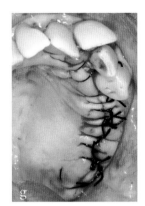

Fig 3-10g (right) Final closure; 3-0 sutures have been used in this case given the need for firm wound closure.

Epulis Excision

Conservative surgical excisional biopsy is the treatment of choice for small lesions with a benign appearance and behaviour, and which do not regress following improved plaque control. The excision should extend down to the periosteum, and adjacent teeth should be thoroughly scaled to remove debris and reduce the likelihood of recurrence. If the lesion radiologically appears to involve bone (e.g. central giant cell granuloma), thorough curettage of the adjacent bone is important to help prevent recurrence, and therefore a minimal mucoperiosteal flap should be raised post-excision, to facilitate thorough bony curettage. Following excision, the gingivae may require recontouring to produce a favourable morphology for oral hygiene practice. For very vascular lesions, use of a local anaesthetic with good vasoconstrictive properties is essential. It may be prudent to have an electrosurgery or diathermy device on hand, to control haemorrhage from a small, severed feeder vessel.

The application of a periodontal dressing is useful as a pressure pack. For definitive diagnosis, histopathological examination is required. It is important that the biopsy tissues are handled carefully to prevent damage that may compromise their diagnostic value.

Wedge Excision

The wedge excision is used to surgically treat periodontal pockets around lone-standing teeth, most often at their distal aspects (the distal wedge excision). The elimination of periodontal pocketing on the distal surfaces of posterior molars may be impeded by fibrous tissue in the tuberosity region or a prominent retromolar pad.

A triangular-shaped incision is made with a scalpel to outline the wedge. The incisions are made down to, and converge at, the alveolar crest. Intrasulcular incisions are made, and a full thickness mucoperiosteal flap raised on the buccal and lingual aspects of the tooth. The wedge can be held with haemostats and then removed by sharp dissection. Root surface debridement may be carried out at this stage. Buccal and lingual flaps are thinned by undermining dissection, if necessary, and then repositioned with securely placed interrupted sutures to eliminate the pocket. Fig 3-11 is a schematic diagram illustrating the distal wedge excision. An alternative approach is illustrated in Fig 3-12 where parallel incisions are made and a distal traversing incision isolates the distal wedge.

Periodontal Dressings

Following procedures that leave a large amount of exposed tissue, or where a pressure pack is deemed necessary to maintain interproximal embrasures in the immediate post-surgical phase, periodontal dressings may be employed. A commonly used periodontal dressing is Coe-Pak (Fig 3-8j), which is a zinc oxide-based formulation. The procedure for its use is outlined below:

- The surgical site is kept dry and free from saliva using suction and damp gauze swabs.
- The Coe-Pak is mixed according to the manufacturer's instructions and handled with lightly vaselined gloves.
- It is rolled into a short, thin roll and then closely adapted to the buccal and lingual surfaces and pressed interdentally with a plastic instrument to gain mechanical retention from embrasure areas.
- Placement of the dressing should not interfere with muscle, cheek or fraenal attachments, because overextension can cause irritation. The occlusion should be checked to ensure it is not impeded during mandibular closure. Care is also needed if a removable prosthesis needs to be inserted over the affected teeth.
- Dressings are usually removed after seven days and a prescription of a desensitising agent for exposed tooth surfaces may be considered at this stage.

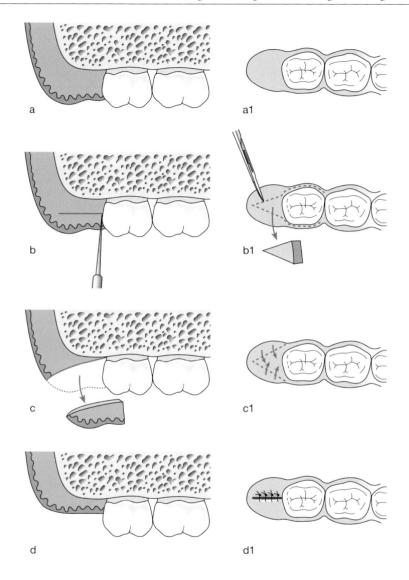

Fig 3-11 Schematic diagram illustrating the distal wedge excision.

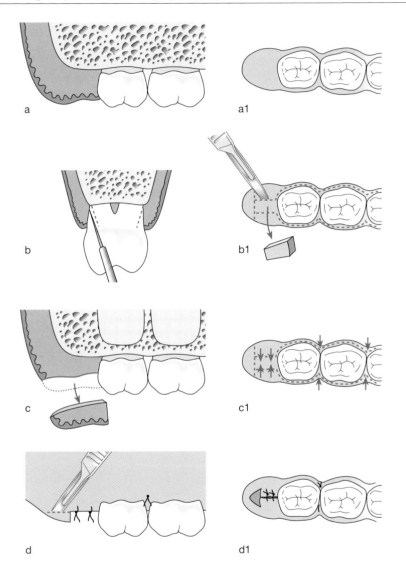

Fig 3-12 Schematic diagram illustrating the distal wedge excision using parallel incisions and distal transverse relieving incision.

Maintenance

Recurrence of drug-induced or hereditary gingival enlargement often arises following surgical management and the patient frequently requires retreatment. It is fundamental to maintain a strict oral hygiene programme. Where poor plaque control has contributed to recurrence, the periodontal surgeon should be wary about embarking upon further surgical treatment.

Further Reading

Chapple ILC, Hamburger J. Periodontal Medicine – A Window on the Body. Chapple ILC (ed). Quintessentials of Dental Practice – 43/44, Periodontology – 5. London: Quintessence Publishing Co. Ltd, 2006.

Mavrogiannis M, Ellis JS, Thomason JM, Seymour RA. The management of drug induced gingival overgrowth. J Clin Periodontol 2006;33:434–439.

Chapter 4

Access Flaps for Surgical Root Surface Debridement

Aim

The aim of the chapter is to review the indications and contraindications for surgical root surface debridement and to discuss the procedure in detail.

Outcome

Having read this chapter, the reader should be able to decide which clinical situations may necessitate surgical access for RSD and have a clear understanding of the procedures involved.

Introduction

Periodontitis is an inflammatory lesion, mediated by host–parasite interactions, that results in loss of connective tissue attachment to the root surface and destruction of adjacent alveolar bone. The disease process initially involves apical migration of the junctional epithelial attachment along the root surface, prior to thickening of the epithelial lining to form an occlusive pocket-lining epithelium.

Suprabony pocketing arises where the apical extent of the pocket is coronal to the alveolar crest; this occurs as a result of horizontal bone loss (Fig 4-1). Infrabony pocketing is where the apical extent of the pocket lies apical to the alveolar crest; this arises normally as a result of vertical bone loss (Fig 4-2).

The choice of treatment for patients with periodontitis varies according to the extent and pattern of attachment loss, local anatomical variations, type of periodontal disease and treatment objectives.

Presurgical Management

All patients should have a comprehensive examination to include radiographic analysis, detailed pocket charting, assessment of furcation status, bleeding on probing, mobility status and presence of suppuration. This information should

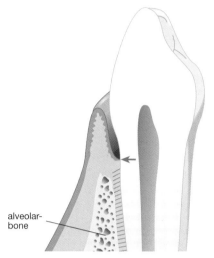

alveolar-
bone

Fig 4-1 Suprabony pocketing.

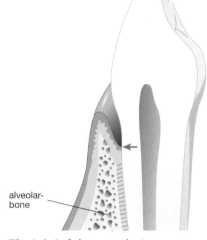

alveolar-
bone

Fig 4-2 Infrabony pocketing.

be recorded at the initial visit and is important for diagnosis, treatment planning and determining prognosis. The same details should be recorded during and after presurgical therapy and surgical treatment as they give an indication of treatment success and may draw attention to specific problems or areas requiring further therapy.

All but the most aggressive forms of periodontitis require an initial phase of non-surgical therapy. This usually includes:
• Patient education in their disease and associated risk factors.
• Rigorous oral hygiene.
• Smoking cessation advice.
• Control of contributing systemic risk factors, e.g. diabetes mellitus.
• Supra- and subgingival scaling and RSD. The objective of scaling and RSD is the complete removal of bacteria, biofilm, endotoxin and calculus to achieve a biologically acceptable root surface.
• Local factors contributing to chronic periodontitis should be removed or controlled. Consideration should be given to carrying out the following:
  – removal of overhanging restoration margins
  – reshaping or replacing over-contoured crowns
  – replacement of poorly designed and fitting removable prostheses

– restoration of carious lesions
– orthodontic treatment
– treatment of occlusal trauma.

Teeth with a poor prognosis, requiring extraction, need to be identified. Extractions of compromised teeth should be carried out expediently to aid the overall treatment plan.

Aggressive Periodontitis

Patients with aggressive forms of periodontitis will usually require referral to specialist services for non-surgical therapy with adjunctive antibiotics. Adjunctive antibiotic therapy is of proven value in the treatment of aggressive periodontitis, which often involves several specific pathogens that have the potential to invade pocket epithelium and connective tissue, and to colonise non-gingival reservoir sites. Where disease is refractory to this approach, surgical intervention may be considered.

Outcomes following scaling and RSD include:
• reduction of clinical inflammation
• microbial shift to a less pathogenic sub-gingival flora
• decreased probing depth
• gain of clinical attachment
• slower disease progression
• gingival recession
• tightening of the gingival cuff and pocket reduction.

Surgical Management

If the results of initial therapy do not control the periodontitis, surgery may be considered. Several factors may limit the effectiveness of non-surgical RSD:
• complex root anatomy
• furcations
• deeper pockets
• patient-specific factors (see Chapter 1).

Surgical access is often necessary to facilitate mechanical instrumentation of the roots. This approach provides direct access to the root surface. Surgical RSD largely involves procedures to improve access for instrumentation and surgical elimination of the pocket to enable the patient to clean to the depth of the sulcus.

Objectives of Surgical Root Surface Debridement
• Improved visibility of the root surface.
• Accessibility for exploration of the root surface and instrumentation.
• Removal of plaque, calculus and other plaque retentive features.
• Elimination of periodontal pockets > 4 mm.
• Creation of a dentogingival morphology to facilitate oral hygiene procedures.
• Allowing placement of regenerative materials (Chapter 5).

A drawback to surgical RSD is the potential for gingival recession. This may lead to dentine hypersensitivity and leave the root surface vulnerable to caries, and may also have implications for aesthetics around anterior teeth. The risk of gingival recession should be discussed thoroughly with the patient prior to any treatment as part of the informed consent process. Indications and contraindications to surgical RSD are listed in Table 4-1.

Table 4-1 **Indications and contraindications to surgical RSD**

Indications	Contraindications
Pocketing ≥ 5 mm with clinical signs of inflammation, which has not resolved using non-surgical methods	Any medical condition that contraindicates surgery
To facilitate placement of regenerative materials	Poor plaque control/motivation
Difficult access to root surfaces	Positive smoking status
	Previous multiple failed attempts

Two commonly used flap designs that allow access for RSD are discussed below and advantages of each technique are shown in Table 4-2.

Simple Replaced Flap (Envelope Flap)
Following administration of local analgesia, an intrasulcular incision is made (Fig 4-3). Occasionally, one or two vertical relieving incisions may be required to allow better access and visibility without placing undue tension upon the flap. A full-thickness mucoperiosteal flap is raised (Fig 4-4). The basic principles of flap design must be followed:

- The flap must be of a sufficient size to expose the relevant underlying anatomy.
- The base must be wide enough to maintain adequate blood supply.
- The incisions must be long enough to allow movement of the flap without undue tension.
- Care must be exercised to avoid important vessels and nerves.

Table 4-2 **Advantages of a simple flap and a modified Widman flap**

Advantages of simple replaced flap	Advantages of modified Widman flap (page 57)
Good access and visualisation of root surfaces and alveolar bone	Close adaptation of soft tissues to the root surfaces
Technically less demanding	Pocket depth can be surgically reduced, if necessary
Less post-operative recession	
Flap may be repositioned coronally or apically	

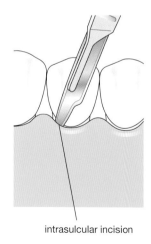

intrasulcular incision

Fig 4-3 Intrasulcular incision.

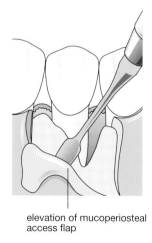

elevation of mucoperiosteal access flap

Fig 4-4 Full-thickness mucoperiosteal flap is raised.

In order to justify a surgical approach to RSD, it is essential to be able to clearly visualise the entire root surface. This requires comprehensive removal of granulation tissue and the use of ultrasonic or sonic scaler instrumentation.

Removal of granulation tissue
Whilst studies have shown that complete granulation tissue removal is not necessary for a successful surgical outcome, the process of thorough removal of granulation tissue radically improves visual access. Granulation tissue bleeds significantly and obscures root surface visualisation. Removal of granulation tissue can be time-consuming and technically demanding as it is frequently very adherent to the root, bone and soft tissues; the use of sharp area-specific curettes is recommended.

Root surface instrumentation
The aim of instrumentation is to allow access to the root surfaces to mechanically disrupt soft subgingival plaque while also removing any adherent mineralised calculus deposits and endotoxin-associated cementum. Good access and visualisation of the root surface are essential and can be improved using magnification loupes or a microscope.

There are a multitude of instruments available for RSD. They are broadly classified into mechanical (ultrasonic or sonic) or hand instruments. Several studies have demonstrated no difference in outcome from utilisation of mechanical or hand instrumentation, or indeed between ultrasonic or sonic instrumentation (Baderston et al., 1981, 1984; Torafson et al., 1979).

Ultrasonic instruments (Fig 4-5) are power-driven instruments of either magnetostrictive or piezoelectric design and which operate at a high frequency above 25 kHz. Their vibrations create turbulence in the microbial colony through "cavitation" and "acoustic microstreaming". Cavitation is the production of air bubbles within the water irrigant, which carry large amounts of potential energy. When the bubbles implode or strike a root surface they release that energy, and this has been shown to destroy endotoxin and bacteria within the biofilm. Acoustic microstreaming is the production of high-pressure currents within the irrigant, which create shear stresses at current interfaces, which in turn damage biofilms and their contents. During ultrasonic instrumentation, as much of the instrument body as possible should be held in contact with the root to avoid grooving or indeed cutting the root surface. Most ultrasonic tips have a straight profile at their tip, making instrumentation of the highly variable morphology of the root difficult. For this reason, and because tactile feedback is poor from mechanical

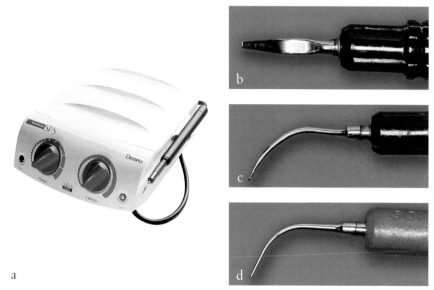

Fig 4-5 (a) Magnetostrictive (Cavitron) scaler manufactured by Dentsply; (b) beavertail tip used for removal of heavy calculus deposits; (c) universal tip used for moderate supra- and subgingival calculus deposits; (d) precision (slimline) tip used to provide best access to deep pockets and furcation areas.

instruments, supplemental hand instrumentation is recommended to establish thorough debridement. Interestingly, studies have shown that utilisation of a half-power setting for ultrasonic scalers is as effective as a full-power setting and less likely to cause root surface damage (Chapple et al., 1995) and that clinical outcomes are comparable whether water or chlorhexidine are used as ultrasonic irrigants (Chapple et al., 1992).

Sonic instruments operate <18 kHz (typically 3–8 kHz) and their pattern of oscillation is different from that of ultrasonic scalers. The differences between these two broad instrument groups are summarised in Table 4-3.

Hand instrumentation is usually carried out using area-specific curettes such as the Gracey curettes (Fig 4-6). These are designed so that each blade adapts to a specific tooth surface or area, and only one cutting edge on each blade is used. Furcation curettes (Fig 4-7) are small curettes designed to fit into

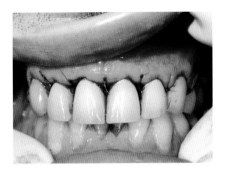

Fig 4-9 Approximation of wound edges with sutures.

tooth down to alveolar bone crest approximately 1 mm from the gingival margin (Fig 4-10). If the pocketing is less than 5 mm or aesthetic considerations are important, the incision may become intrasulcular in localised areas. A mucoperiosteal flap is reflected within the attached gingivae to allow vision of the root surface. Flap elevation is therefore limited. An intrasulcular incision is made to the depth of the pocket; this helps to release the resultant tissue collar (Fig 4-11). A third, horizontal incision may be

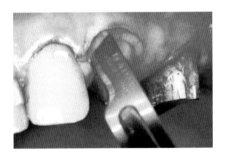

Fig 4-10 Scalloped inverse bevel incision. (Courtesy of Sato, *Periodontal Surgery: A Clinical Atlas*, 2000)

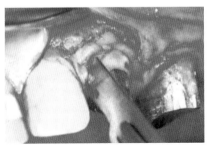

Fig 4-11 Intrasulcular incision to release tissue collar. (Courtesy of Sato, *Periodontal Surgery: A Clinical Atlas*, 2000)

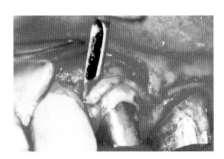

Fig 4-12 Horizontal incision to separate the soft tissue collar from the bone. (Courtesy of Sato, *Periodontal Surgery: A Clinical Atlas,* 2000)

required to separate the soft tissue collar from the bone (Fig 4-12), although most periodontal surgeons would utilise a sharp curette for this purpose. Following debridement, the flap is replaced with simple, interrupted sutures and full coverage of interproximal bone is ensured. This technique reduces the preoperative pocket depth.

The distal wedge excision is used to surgically treat periodontal pockets around lone-standing teeth, most often at their distal aspects. This technique has been described in Chapter 3.

Suturing
An illustration of how to perform the simple interrupted suture is shown in Figure 4-13 and the technique is described below:

1. The needle is passed through the buccal flap approximately 3 mm from the gingival margin.
2. It is then passed through the palatal/lingual flap, again approximately 3 mm from the gingival margin.
3. The needle is passed through the interdental space without piercing tissue and brought back to the buccal side.
4. The long end of the suture is passed twice around the needle holders and then the short end grasped with the tips of the holders and drawn through the loops.
5. To complete a second knot, the long end of the suture is wound once around the needle holders in a reverse direction, the short end is pulled through and the knot is completed. Some suture materials are very smooth and therefore require an extra turn or two so the knots do not unravel.
6. The suture ends are cut approximately 3 mm from the knot.

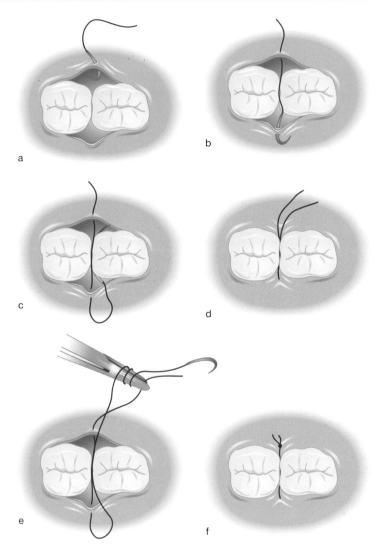

Fig 4-13 A sequence illustrating the simple interrupted suture.

The Use of a Periodontal Pressure Dressing

Periodontal dressings such as Coe-Pak may be used to fill embrasure spaces and allow close adaptation of the flap in the immediate post-operative period (see Chapters 2 and 3); they prevent a proliferative healing response that may close up interdental spaces and thereby compromise access for home care.

Post-operative Instructions

It is vital that patients are given comprehensive post-operative instructions both verbally and in the form of a written sheet that they may take with them.

These should include:
• Not brushing the operative site for seven days.
• The use of a 0.2% chlorhexidine mouthwash to facilitate plaque control during the period of non-brushing.
• Instructions on how to manage a post-operative bleed.
• Pain control (analgesia).

Review

The patient should be seen one week post-operatively to review healing, for suture removal and removal of any surgical dressings. It is vital at this appointment to perform a thorough professional prophylaxis and instruct patients in gentle brushing, building up to full pressure after a further five to seven days. The chlorhexidine mouthwash should be stopped at this point. Pockets should not be probed until at least eight weeks following surgery as earlier probing may disrupt the early stages of healing.

Periodontal Maintenance

A long-term recall programme is necessary to evaluate the success of therapy. Patients should be reviewed at regular intervals to monitor plaque control and allow early detection of recurrent disease. Detailed recording of pocket depths around all tooth surfaces is essential to detect bleeding from the base of pockets, and, if necessary, attachment levels should be evaluated where recession is evident. With this approach, recurrent disease may be identified in a site-specific manner early and simple corrective measures implemented non-surgically.

Key Points

• The aim of surgical RSD is to reduce probing pocket depths and restore gingival contours to a condition that can be easily maintained by the patient.
• Surgical RSD should only be performed when non-surgical therapy has failed to produce adequate healing in patients with a high standard of home care.

References

Ramfjord SP, Nissle RR. The modified Widman flap. J Periodontol 1974;45:601–607.

Baderston A, Nilveus R, Egelberg J. Effect of nonsurgical therapy I: moderately advanced periodontitis. J Clin Periodontal 1981;8:57–72.

Baderston A, Nilveus R, Egelberg J. Effect of nonsurgical therapy II: severely advanced periodontitis. J Clin Periodontal 1984;11:63–76.

Chapple ILC, Walmsley AD, Saxby MS, Moscrop H. Effect of subgingival irrigation with chlorhexidine during ulstrasonic scaling. J Periodontol 1992;63:812–816.

Chapple ILC, Walmsley AD, Saxby MS, Moscrop H. Effect of instrument power setting during ulstrasonic scaling upon treatment outcome. J Periodontal 1995;66: 756–760.

Rosling B, Nyman S, Lindh J. The effect of systematic plaque control on bone regeneration in infrabony pockets. J Clin Periodontal 1976;3:38–53.

Torfason T, Kiger R, Selvig KA, Egelberg J. Clinical improvement of gingival conditions following ultrasonic versus hand instrumentation of periodontal pockets. J Clin Periodontal 1979;6:165–176.

Further Reading

Silverstein LH, Christensen GJ. Principles of dental suturing: the complete guide to surgical closure. Mahwah NJ: Montage Media Corporation, 1999.

Wang HL, Greenwell H. Surgical periodontal therapy. Periodontol 2000, 2001;25:89–99.

Chapter 5
Regenerative Periodontal Techniques

Aim

This chapter aims to provide a historical overview of the principles underlying guided periodontal tissue regeneration (GTR) and to illustrate the different surgical techniques that may be employed to regenerate lost periodontal tissues. It will allude to the limited evidence base for efficacy of some of these techniques and also demonstrate the core principles, which may also be applied to guided bone regeneration (GBR).

Outcome

Having read this chapter, the reader should be familiar with the biological basis for, and principles underlying, GTR and, most importantly, be conversant with their limitations, indications and contraindications.

Introduction

Immediately following non-surgical or surgical RSD, the pocket space and connective tissues lying adjacent to the root surface are occupied by a thin blood clot. The principles of wound healing follow those for secondary intention healing, in that the clot initially "organises" and is then replaced by fibrous repair tissue. The pioneering research of Tony Melcher in the 1960s and 1970s led to the classic paradigm that "the first cells to repopulate a root surface will dictate the nature and quality of tissue that forms there" (Melcher, 1976). Of those cell types that have the potential to repopulate the postoperative wound, the fastest dividing cells are the oral epithelial cells (Fig 5-1), and hence the majority of new root surface attachment formed is epithelial in nature – the aptly named long junctional epithelium (LJE) (Caton et al., 1980).

The classical biological processes that contribute to pocket-depth reduction post-therapy are:
• LJE formation (one week)
• Resolution of gingival inflammation (two weeks)

- Remodelling of the gingival connective tissues and subsequent shrinkage owing to collagen maturation by cross-linkage (two to three months).

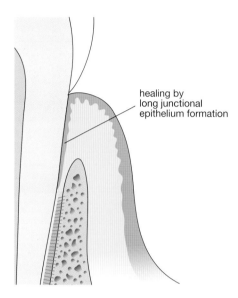

healing by
long junctional
epithelium formation

Fig 5-1 Longitudinal section of treated pocket, demonstrating formation of a new long junctional epithelial attachment to the treated root surface.

Hence, reprobing within three months of therapy is generally not recommended. Despite the LJE formation, Rosling et al. (1976) demonstrated that new bone will also form at the base of infrabony defects (Fig 5-2a,b).

Despite this, histological studies have demonstrated that epithelium may be interposed between the new alveolar bone and root surface in such cases (Caton and Greenstein, 1993). Classical periodontal regeneration, however, requires the formulation of a new connective tissue attachment to the root surface, achieved by selectively guiding undifferentiated stem cells from the periodontal ligament and adjacent alveolar bone to repopulate a treated root surface. This process should lead to new cementum formation, followed by new periodontal ligament and adjacent alveolar bone formation. True periodontal regeneration should also recreate the overlying gingival epithelium and connective tissues; this is, however, not yet technically possible. This latter failure is crucial to understanding the limitations of contemporary GTR, because complete periodontal regeneration is rarely achieved and thus recession is a component of healing even post-GTR in the "real world". It is important that patients are advised of this as part of the informed consent process.

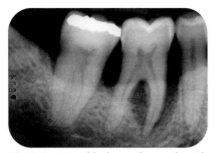 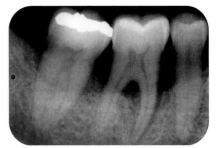

Fig 5-2a Mandibular molar tooth with furcation involvement and bone loss close to the apex of the mesial root pre-non-surgical RSD.

Fig 5-2b The same tooth as in Fig 5-2a, 12 months following non-surgical RSD. Note the bony infill at the base of the vertical bone defect (whether an epithelial layer exists between the root surface and the new bone in this case is unknown).

Whilst the LJE is relatively stable, it is far less robust than the original periodontal connective tissue attachment and hence supportive care programmes involving regular (3–4 monthly) recalls for professional reinforcement of oral hygiene and professional prophylaxis remain the mainstay of successful traditional periodontal therapies. The ultimate goal of periodontal therapy is to replace the supporting apparatus that has been destroyed by the disease process with cells and tissues identical to those that were lost – this is true regeneration.

Terminology

Repair – is the restoration of new tissue that does not replicate the structure and function of the lost tissues (Melcher, 1969).

Regeneration – is the biological process by which the architecture and function of the lost tissue is completely restored (Melcher, 1969).

Connective tissue re-attachment – is the reunion of connective tissue with a root surface on which a viable periodontal ligament exists, for example following a surgical flap for peri-radicular surgery where there was *no* underlying periodontal disease (Isidor, 1985).

Connective tissue new attachment – is the union of connective tissue with a root surface that has been deprived of its periodontal ligament (Isidor, 1985).

It is important to appreciate that a new attachment may be formed by epithelium (new epithelial attachment) or by connective tissue (new connective tissue attachment) and it is the latter that GTR aims to achieve.

Biological Principles Underpinning GTR

The dentogingival anatomy immediately post-therapy, with a blood clot sitting adjacent to the debrided root surface, is illustrated in Fig 5-3. The natural history of healing is that the oral epithelial cells migrate onto the root surface and attach via hemi-desmosomal junctions to form the LJE. If the epithelial down-growth is blocked using a physical barrier then the next cell type to reach the root surface would be the gingival fibroblasts and the connective tissues they form. The gingival connective tissues are dynamic, and collagen replacement is affected by collagenase production by gingival fibroblasts. In areas where the RSD has denuded the root surface of cementum, the liberation of collagenases may resorb the root dentine organic matrix, thus creating external root resorption (Fig 5-4). This is undesirable; therefore any barrier membrane should also isolate the cleaned root surface

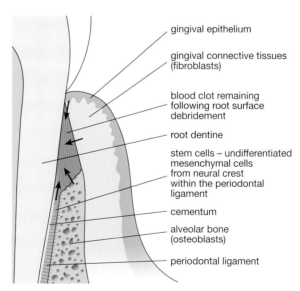

Fig 5-3 Longitudinal section of treated pocket, demonstrating (by arrows) the cells with the potential to colonise the root surface. The oral epithelial cells are the first to reach the root surface, forming a new long junctional epithelial attachment at the coronal aspect.

from the gingival connective tissues, thereby leaving two remaining potential sources of cells to re-populate the wound:

- osteoblasts from the adjacent bone
- undifferentiated stem cells (derived from the embryonal neural crest) within the periodontal ligament (PDL).

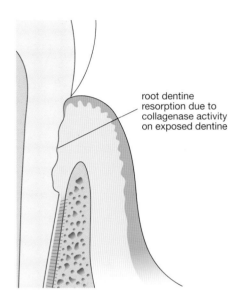

root dentine resorption due to collagenase activity on exposed dentine

Fig 5-4 If the oral epithelium is physically blocked from reaching the treated root surface, the next cells to contact are those of the gingival connective tissues. Collagenases produced by gingival fibroblasts were shown in animal models to resorb the root surface where denuded of cementum by instrumentation.

Osteoclasts are more slowly dividing than the PDL stem cells; therefore it is largely academic to speculate as to what their contact with the root surface would achieve. In experimental models it was demonstrated that the collagenases produced by osteocytes/clasts within bone resorbed the root dentine (as with the gingival connective tissues), and since bone is a dynamic and vital tissue, bony ingress to the resorbed dentine spaces arose. The result was ankylosis (Fig 5-5), an undesirable outcome for natural teeth, but a very desirable one for titanium implants, where the term "osseointegration" is now employed to describe the resulting tight union between bone and the implant surface.

The potential for periodontal tissue regeneration was demonstrated in a series of elegant histological studies (Nyman et al., 1982). Following surgical flap procedures, a buccal and approximal bone window was created; all exposed

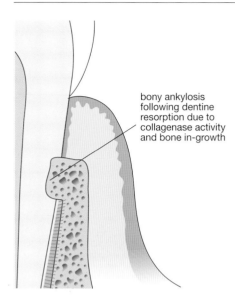

bony ankylosis
following dentine
resorption due to
collagenase activity
and bone in-growth

Fig 5-5 In animal models, where bone was allowed to reach the root surface, resorption also took place (as with Fig 5-4), but new bone formed into resorption lacunae, creating an ankylosis.

cementum was then curetted prior to placement of a 0.22 mm Millipore filter over the buccal fenestration and flap closure. Six months later, new cementum with inserting connective tissue fibres had formed, alongside significant (up to 3.9 mm) bone growth. A further study utilised Millipore and Goretex filters placed over surgically induced defects, where cementum was denuded from non-periodontitis affected roots (Gottlow et al., 1984). Six months later, and after exposure to long-term plaque accumulation, block dissected biopsies demonstrated new cementum formation with new PDL fibre insertion. Nyman and colleagues (1982) also demonstrated new cementum and bone formation around a human mandibular incisor with advanced periodontitis in a 47-year-old male, using a Millipore filter and the now standard surgically induced root surface notch as a reference point from which to measure new connective tissue attachment.

Subsequent studies (e.g. Gottlow et al., 1986) demonstrated that the surgical placement of a barrier membrane made from Goretex (expanded polytetrafluoroethylene – ePTFE) fibres tied around the cervical margin of the tooth and draped beneath a mucoperiosteal flap and onto the alveolar bone surface (Fig 5-6) was capable of preventing both the down-growth of oral epithelial cells and the trans-growth of gingival fibroblasts onto the cleaned root surface. The result was that undifferentiated stem cells from the PDL

Fig 5-6 The placement of an ePTFE membrane. The open micropore surface is designed to slow down the migration of large (relative to fibroblasts) epithelial cells. The occlusive "skirt" draped over the alveolus had a smaller micropore structure designed to prevent slender gingival fibroblasts from traversing the membrane onto the root surface.

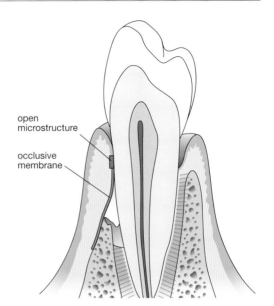

migrated into the wound, and sequential differentiation into cementoblasts and fibroblasts led to the formation of new cementum and new PDL fibres inserting into new alveolar bone (Fig 5-7). These studies established the principles of periodontal regeneration and verified Melcher's theories; GTR was born, and the benefits of stem cell biology were realised for the first time in periodontology.

Surgical Planning for Membrane GTR

Indications
- Most Class II furcations.
- Early Class III furcations.
- Two- or three-walled bony defects.
- Circumferential "moat defects".

Contraindications
- Poor oral hygiene – failure more likely.
- Patient attitude, e.g. expectations, compliance – technically challenging procedures.
- Economics – expensive.
- Multiple infrabony defects – cost, time and logistics.

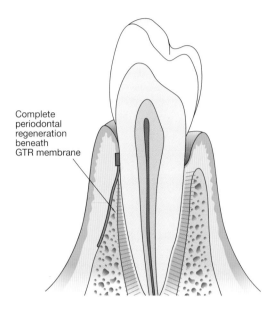

Complete
periodontal
regeneration
beneath
GTR membrane

Fig 5-7 An illustration of "theoretical" complete regeneration following Goretex membrane placement. In reality at six weeks, when membranes were removed, the regenerated tissue was a red gelatinous tissue which did not resemble architecturally the definitive regenerated structures: this process takes approximately 12 months.

- Class III furcation defects – owing to a failure of coronal bone growth.
- One-walled bony defects – owing to a lack of vertical bony walls to supply osteoblasts.
- Horizontal bone loss – coronal bone growth did not occur.
- Lack of soft tissue to cover space coronally – membrane exposure, plaque accumulation and recession.
- Smoking.
- Medical history.

What Went Wrong in Practice and Why?

The majority of membranes became exposed between the first surgical stage and their surgical removal six weeks later. Many claimed this did not arise in their cases, but those with experience recognised that this was either "luck" or due to the fact that those operators had not performed a sufficient number of procedures to justify authoritative comment! Exposure was simply because the ePTFE membranes were literally "non-stick" and there was no initial fibrinous union between the adjacent flap and membrane surface; thus muscular pull from the circum-oral musculature drew the flap apically and exposed membranes, resulting in recession. Other complications included:

- any complications for routine flap surgery
- failure of procedure
- additional therapy needed, so costly
- infection/abscess formation
- exfoliation of graft/membrane
- oral hygiene modifications always needed
- membrane exposure due to trauma, e.g. caused by brushing
- prolonged post-operative management
- pulpitis due to furcation cleaning
- resulting gingival architecture poor for cleaning
- aesthetic compromise – must warn patient
- hypersensitivity
- potential for rapid recurrence of defect
- long-term maintenance essential.

Objectives of GTR surgery
- disease arrestment
- regain optimal health, function, aesthetics
- regeneration where feasible
- maintenance of health.

Criteria for Success
- absence of bleeding to probe
- establishing a non-destructive microbiota
- improvement in attachment level
- ease of maintenance.

The Need for Two-stage Surgery
The non-resorbable Goretex membranes required a second surgical incision (intrasulcular) to expose them and facilitate removal (Figs 5-7, 5-8). This exposed regenerated marginal tissues and resulted in some loss of new attachment.

Case Selection and Planning
Given the costs and surgical skill necessary, these procedures were limited to strategically important teeth, such as the bridge abutment in Fig 5-9a.

The Surgical Phase
A Goretex procedure is illustrated in Fig 5-9b–g. Following elevation of a mucoperiosteal flap over sound bone margins, the defect was debrided thoroughly. A space maintainer was packed over the root surface and a

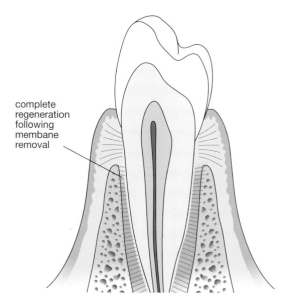

complete
regeneration
following
membane
removal

Fig 5-8 Following membrane removal at six weeks, the immature "gelatinous" tissue that formed beneath the membrane reorganised ultimately to a new connective tissue attachment. Complete regeneration beneath the ePTFE membrane was the theoretical ideal, and did sometimes occur.

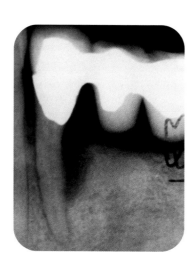

Fig 5-9a Preoperative radiograph of a mandibular left first premolar, with a distal two-walled vertical bone defect. This tooth was strategically important as the mesial abutment to a fixed–fixed bridge (the distal abutment was the mandibular left second molar). If lost, the bridge would have been lost and a removable partial denture or implant-retained prosthesis required.

template used to cut the membrane to size. The definitive membrane was positioned to cover the defect, so that its margins lay over sound bone, and was secured with a sling suture around the neck of the tooth. The flap was then closed with monofilament Goretex simple interrupted sutures.

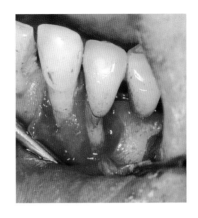

Fig 5-9b A two-sided full-thickness muco-periosteal flap was raised to provide clear access to the defect, which had developed owing to a dilacerated root creating a "V-shaped" defect at the crown–root interface. This was thoroughly debrided (Chapter 4) using ultrasonic and hand instrumentation and the patient counselled (specific oral hygiene instruction) about why the defect had developed, to prevent its recurrence post-surgery.

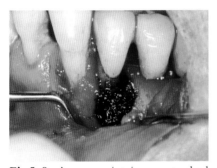

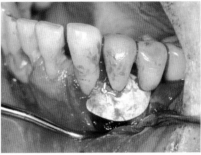

Fig 5-9c A space maintainer was packed into the defect. The biomaterial used was a resorbable Surgicel haemostatic pack. Evidence that such packs inhibited osteogenesis emerged from the literature at a later date, and therefore use of such agents for defect packing ceased.

Fig 5-9d A Goretex ePTFE membrane is adapted over the defect. Note the membrane does not fully cover the inferior margin of the bone defect and therefore had to be readapted to do so prior to flap closure.

Fig 5-9e Simple interrupted sutures are used to close the flap (see Fig 4-13). Goretex ePTFE monofilament sutures were used in this case as they were non-irritant, non-plaque-retentive and could be left in place to prevent apical flap displacement for the full six weeks until second-stage surgery for membrane removal.

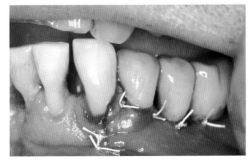

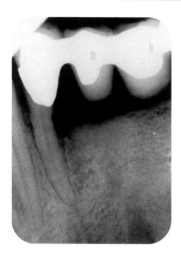

Fig 5-9f A radiograph at six months post-GTR surgery demonstrates substantial bone regeneration.

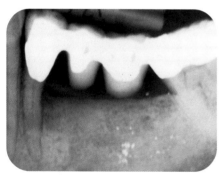

Fig 5-9g A radiograph at 12 months demonstrates virtual total regeneration. This situation remains the case at the time of this book going to press – some 15 years later.

Post-operative Care
Patients were advised to refrain from brushing the region for six weeks, and chlorhexidine was used for chemical plaque control. The Goretex sutures were tissue-biocompatible, and as monofilaments did not accumulate plaque or debris; they were therefore left in place for six weeks to prevent recession and membrane exposure until second-phase surgery (membrane removal).

The Outcome of GTR
The definitive outcomes of GTR surgery cannot be determined radiographically until 12 months post-surgery and are variable, between total (Fig 5-9g) and partial (Fig 5-10a,b) regeneration.

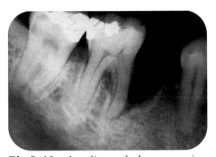

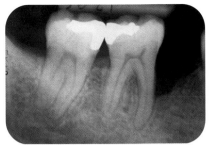

Fig 5-10a A radiograph demonstrating a one-walled vertical bone defect close to the apex of the lower right mandibular molar tooth. This situation (one-walled defect) is not suited to GTR.

Fig 5-10b A radiograph of the tooth in Fig 5-10a, 12 months post-surgery, demonstrating partial bone regeneration, despite the unfavourable anatomy.

Modifications to the Original Membranes

A modification to the original Goretex ePTFE membranes utilised titanium reinforcement spines, fabricated in different geometric patterns for periodontal and implant membranes. This facilitated "tenting" of the membrane over the defect/blood clot to maintain the space, into which regeneration occurred, without the need to pack a space maintainer beneath the membranes (Fig 5-11).

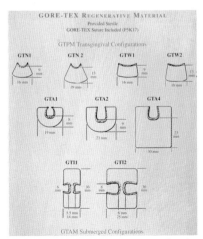

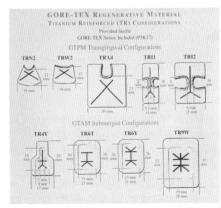

Fig 5-11 Examples of shapes of traditional non-reinforced and titanium-reinforced Goretex membranes.

Resorbable GTR membranes

A variety of resorbable membranes followed the original Goretex ePTFE membranes, with the advantage of one-stage surgery (no need for membrane removal), which prevented exposure of immature regenerated tissues at the time of membrane removal. Examples included membranes comprising:

- polyglycolide co-polymers such as Vicryl membranes (Ethicon)
- poly-DL lactide (e.g. "Atrisorb" by Atrix Lab. Inc), Poly-D, L lactide/ ATBC (acetyltributyl citrate – Guidor by Guidor, Huddinge, Sweden)
- oxidised cellulose
- collagen/polylactic acid (e.g. Bio-Gide, Geistlich)
- cargile
- polylactic/polyglyclic acid ("Resolut" by WL Gore & Associates, Inc.).

A resorbable Vicryl membrane is shown in Fig 5-12, and Fig 5-13 shows pre- and post-surgical radiographs following GTR using Vicryl to a mandibular left canine.

Systematic reviews of randomised controlled trials reporting the use of both non-resorbable and resorbable membranes have been reported for infrabony and furcation defects (Needleman et al., 2002; Jepsen et al., 2002). Whilst

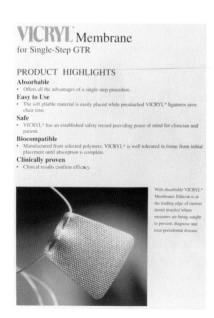

VICRYL Membrane
for Single-Step GTR

PRODUCT HIGHLIGHTS

Absorbable
- Offers all the advantages of a single-step procedure.

Easy to Use
- The soft pliable material is easily placed while preattached VICRYL* ligatures save chair time.

Safe
- VICRYL* has an established safety record providing peace of mind for clinician and patient.

Biocompatible
- Manufactured from selected polymers. VICRYL* is well tolerated in tissue from initial placement until absorption is complete.

Clinically proven
- Clinical results confirm efficacy.

With absorbable VICRYL* Membranes Ethicon is at the leading edge of current dental practice where measures are being sought to prevent, diagnose and treat periodontal disease.

Fig 5-12 A resorbable Vicryl membrane with prethreaded suture, for one-stage GTR surgery.

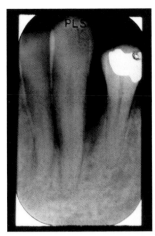 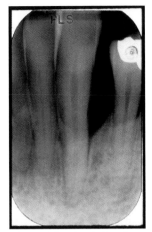

Fig 5-13a A defect around a mandibular canine prior to GTR using a resorbable Vicryl membrane.

Fig 5-13b The defect from Fig 5-13a 12 months post-surgery, demonstrating some improvement in bone density and bone levels.

both reviews reported statistically significant improvements from the use of GTR membranes over open-flap debridement, improvements were modest at best and heterogeneity between studies was so large that conclusions regarding clinical rather than statistical benefits were limited.

Enamel Matrix Proteins (Emdogain)

An elegant series of studies by Hammarström and colleagues in the 1990s demonstrated that enamel matrix proteins, purified from porcine tooth germs, had regenerative potential when applied during flap surgery to a root surface that had been treated by open RSD following periodontitis. The epithelial rests of Malassez (from Hertwig's root sheath) in the embryonic tooth germ are known to release enamel matrix proteins, which appear to induce cementoblast formation from undifferentiated mesenchymal stem cells within the periodontal ligament (Hammarström et al., 1997) (Fig 5-14a,b). The suggested sequence of biological events that leads to periodontal attachment formation within the tooth embryo are:

- odontoblasts form mantle dentine matrix
- mantle dentine mineralises
- enamel-related proteins secreted by cells of the epithelial root sheath

number of clinical studies, and these were reviewed by Sculean and Jepsen (2004b). A systematic review by Esposito and colleagues (2004) employed a meta-analysis of eight clinical trials and demonstrated that EMD resulted in an additional 1.3 mm of attachment gain and 1 mm of probing pocket depth (PPD) reduction over open-flap surgical RSD alone, and that there was no evidence of important differences between EMD therapy and membrane GTR.

The main advantage of EMD is its simplicity (Fig 5-16a–c): the lack of adverse events and the fact that it only lengthens open RSD procedures by a few minutes. The disadvantages are those of other regenerative therapies, namely cost and a lack of predictability.

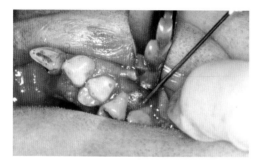

Fig 5-16a Application of EMD during open RSD procedure to a debrided and conditioned root surface. It is useful to keep some EMD gel back to re-inject into the treated pocket after the flap has been replaced and sutured.

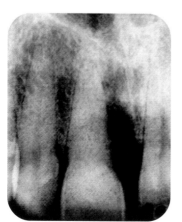

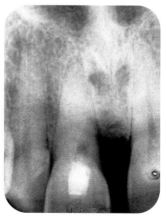

Fig 5-16b Radiograph of infrabony defect mesial to a right maxillary incisor prior to EMD surgery.

Fig 5-16c Radiograph demonstrating the resulting tissue regeneration 12 months following EMD application for the same tooth as in Fig 5-16b.

Bone Grafting and Bioceramic Bone Substitutes

A large number of bone grafting techniques and materials have been developed over the years to facilitate periodontal regeneration. These were very nicely reviewed by Sculean and Jepsen (2004a). In broad terms, there are four main categories of bone substitute:

- Autografts – autogenous bone marrow is collected from one site in an individual and used to graft into a distant site in the same patient. The most common donor site extra-orally is the iliac crest (hip) and intra-orally the chin (via a bone window) or retro-molar area.
- Allografts – allogenic graft materials are those transferred from one member of a species to another genetically dissimilar member of the same species. The most commonly reported allografts are:
  FDBA – mineralised freeze dried bone allografts
  DFDBA – decalcified freeze dried bone allografts.
- Xenografts – these are grafts taken from a donor of a different species from the recipient, e.g. "BioOss" (Geistlich), from the mineral portion of bovine bone.
- Alloplastic biomaterials – these are biocompatible synthetic inorganic materials. Most are resorbable and some have been shown to be osteo-inductive and to inhibit oral epithelial down-growth (e.g. the bioactive glasses). Examples include:
  Hydroxyapatite – both non-resorbable and resorbable forms exist
  Polylactic acid – a resorbable biomaterial
  Bio-active glasses – may be resorbable or non-resorbable and examples include "BioGran" (Orthovita – Figs 5-17 and 5-18a–c) and Perio-glass (NovaBone Products).

Whilst there is some evidence from human histological studies for periodontal regeneration resulting from bovine-derived xenografts, DFDBA and autogenous bone, the reported gains in attachment are modest and there is no evidence of regeneration reported for alloplastic materials in periodontal regeneration (Sculean and Jepsen, 2004a).

Cocktail Procedures

Various "cocktails" of periodontal regenerative methods have been reported, combining, for example, membrane GTR with bioceramic materials or EMD. Data on their benefits are limited in nature and there is no robust evidence that they offer clinically significant advantages over monotherapies.

81

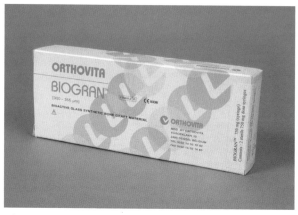

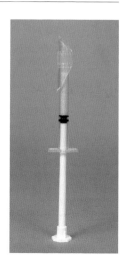

Fig 5-17 An example of a bio-active ceramic alloplastic material.

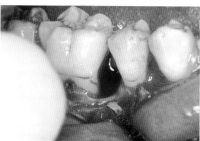

Fig 5-18a Open RSD is performed on the right mandibular first molar after raising a simple replaced mucoperiosteal flap.

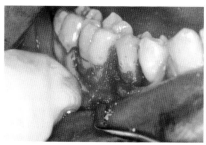

Fig 5-18b BioOss is packed into the debrided surgical defect in the case from 5-18a.

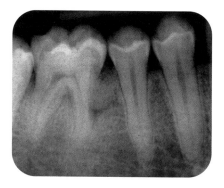

Fig 5-18c Radiological appearance of the case in 5-18b, immediately post-surgery.

Growth Factors

Studies continue into periodontal tissue regeneration using a variety of growth factors such as:
- PDGF – platelet-derived growth factor
- IGF-1 – insulin-like growth factor
- FGF – fibroblast growth factor
- TGFß – transforming growth factor beta
- BMPs – bone morphogenic proteins.

BMP-2 to BMP-9 belong to the TGFß super family of growth factors and recombinant BMP-2, 3 and 7 have been used to regenerate periodontal tissue in animal models. Such growth factors have great potential, but currently remain largely experimental in nature.

Guided Bone Regeneration

The GTR techniques described previously may also be used in periodontal surgery for GBR in certain situations. Examples include:
- Immediately post-extraction to preserve bone prior to implant placement.
- Pre-implant ridge augmentation (Chapter 10).
- In bone regeneration following cyst enucleation (or similar intra-osseous pathology).
- In the management of peri-implantitis – to regenerate bone following implant disinfection.

The most widely used methods for bone regeneration involve resorbable membranes with/without the use of autogenous bone, bone allografts or alloplastic materials, placed beneath the membrane to maintain space into which regeneration takes place following osseoinduction.

The importance of maintaining marginal alveolar bone during surgical exodontia prior to membrane placement is illustrated in Fig 5-19a–d, and Fig 5-20a–c illustrates the re-creation of a canine eminence 18 months post-extraction, prior to implant surgery.

The results of using a xenograft mixed with a local delivery antibiotic (Dentomycin) and placed beneath a resorbable membrane to decontaminate an implant and stimulate bone regeneration, following enucleation of an infected peri-implant cyst, are illustrated in Fig 5-21a–e (page 86).

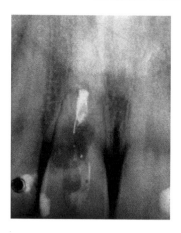

Fig 5-19a A resorbing right maxillary canine which requires extraction.

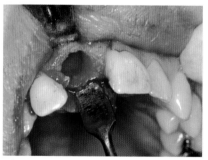

Fig 5-19b The surgical extraction avoids marginal bone removal from socket by careful use of elevators to remove the apical root third.

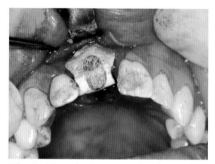

Fig 5-19c A Goretex Oval implant membrane with central open micropore structure.

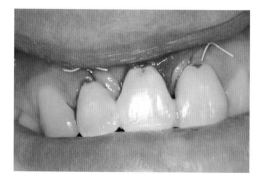

Fig 5-19d Post-surgery from Fig 5-19b–c, a fraenectomy was also performed and the three-sided flap coronally advanced to achieve complete closure. The patient's own crown was used as a temporary adhesive bridge.

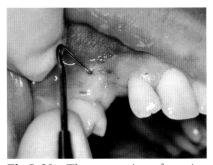

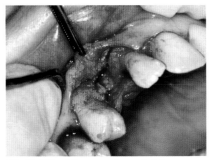

Fig 5-20a The preparation of a canine eminence prior to implant placement in the maxillary right canine region. Horizontal "bone sounding" is being performed using a straight sharp probe under analgesia to determine the bone margins.

Fig 5-20b The case from 5-20a – note the socket is filled with soft tissue which requires removal. The socket wall is perforated internally with a small burr to create bleeding points prior to membrane placement.

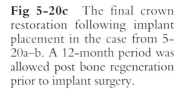

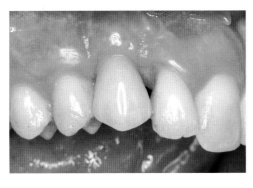

Fig 5-20c The final crown restoration following implant placement in the case from 5-20a–b. A 12-month period was allowed post bone regeneration prior to implant surgery.

There is some evidence that bone regeneration is more predictable than periodontal regeneration, where complete wound closure is achieved over the membrane – that is, in the absence of teeth or a transmucosal implant abutment. This is likely to be due to the fact that healing can occur in the absence of chronic irritation from a plaque biofilm. Therefore, when treating peri-implant bone loss, the transmucosal component is removed and a cover screw used to hold the membrane in place, prior to complete flap closure over the cover screw to re-cover the implant. Resorbable bone screws and pins may also be used to secure the membrane peripherally (Chapter 10).

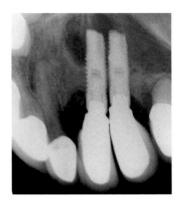

Fig 5-21a Radiograph of peri-implant cyst pre-surgery.

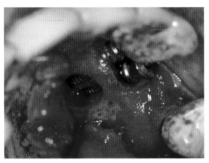

Fig 5-21b Operative site post-enucleation of infected cyst and implant debridement.

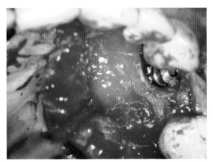

Fig 5-21c The defect packed with BioOss mixed with Dentamycin antibiotic gel.

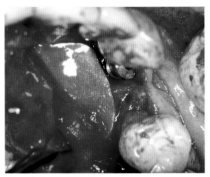

Fig 5-21d BioOss covered with Bio-Gide membrane prior to wound closure.

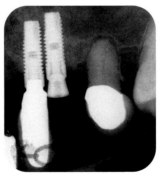

Fig 5-21e The implants from 5-21a, 12 months following regeneration surgery. The implants had re-osseointegrated and were stable.

Key Points

- Case selection is crucial for GTR success.
- Limit use to strategically important teeth, owing to the heterogeneity of results.
- If using membranes, warn patients about recession and membrane exposure.
- There is no robust data to support the use of one method rather than another.
- Use of monofilament sutures reduces plaque accumulation post-surgery.
- Rigorous post-operative care is necessary.

References

Caton J, Nyman S, Zander H. Histometric evaluation of periodontal surgery. II. Connective tissue attachment levels after four regenerative procedures. J Clin Periodontol 1980;7:224–231.

Caton J, Greenstein G. Factors related to periodontal regeneration. Periodontol 2000, 1993;1:9–15.

Esposito M, Coulthard P, Thomsen P, Worthington H. Enamel matrix derivative for periodontal tissue regeneration in treatment of intrabony defects: A Cochrane systematic review. J Dent Educ 2004;68:834–844.

Gottlow J, Nyman S, Karring T, Lindhe J. New attachment formation as a result of controlled tissue regeneration. J Clin Periodontol 1984;11:494–503.

Gottlow J, Nyman S, Lindhe J, Karring T, Wennström J. New attachment formation in human periodontium by guided tissue regeneration. J Clin Periodontol 1986;13:604–616.

Hammarström L. Enamel matrix, cementum development and regeneration. J Clin Periodontol 1997;24:658–668.

Hammarström L, Heijl L, Gestrelius S. Periodontal regeneration in a buccal dehiscence model in monkeys after application of enamel matrix proteins. J Clin Periodontol 1997;24:669–677.

Isidor F, Karring T, Nyman S, Lindhe J. New attachment – reattachment following reconstructive periodontal surgery. J Clin Periodontol 1985;12:728–735.

Jepsen S, Eberhard J, Herrera D, Needleman I. A systematic review of guided tissue regeneration for periodontal furcations defects. What is the effect of guided tissue regeneration compared with surgical debridement in the treatment of furcation defects. J Clin Periodontol 2002;29 (suppl 3):103–116.

Melcher AH. Healing of wounds in the periodontium. In: Melcher AH, Bowen WH (eds). Biology of the Periodontium. London: Academic Press, 1969:497–529.

Melcher AH. On the repair potential of periodontal tissues. J Periodontol 1976;47: 256–260.

Needleman I, Tucker R, Geidrys-Leeper E, Worthington H. A systematic review of guided tissue regeneration for periodontal infrabony defects. J Periodont Res 2002;37:380–388.

Nyman S, Gottlow J, Karring T, Lindhe J. The regenerative potential of the periodontal ligament: an experimental study in the monkey. J Clin Periodontol 1982;9:257–265.

Nyman S, Lindhe J, Karring T, Rylander H. New attachment following surgical treatment of human periodontal disease. J Clin Periodontol 1982;9:290–296.

Rosling B, Nyman S, Lindhe J. The effect of systematic plaque control on bone regeneration in infrabony pockets. J Clin Periodontol 1976;3:38–53.

Sculean A, Jepsen S. Biomaterials for the reconstructive treatment of periodontal intrabony defects. Part 1. Bone grafts and bone substitutes. Perio 2004a;1:5–15.

Sculean A, Jepsen S. Biomaterials for the reconstructive treatment of periodontal intrabony defects. Part II. Guided tissue regeneration, biological agents and combination therapies. Perio 2004b;1:97–109.

Trombelli L, Heitz-Mayfield LJA, Needleman I, Moles D, Scabbia A. A systematic review of graft materials and biological agents for periodontal intraosseous defects. J Clin Periodontol 2002;29:117–135.

Further Reading

Sato N (ed). Periodontal Surgery: A Clinical Atlas. Chicago, London: Quintessence, 2000.

Chapter 6
Periradicular Surgery

Aim

This chapter aims to provide the reader with guidance on case selection and a step-by-step approach to contemporary techniques used in periradicular surgery.

Outcome

Having read this chapter the reader will be aware of contemporary techniques used in periradicular surgery.

Introduction

"Periradicular surgery" is the contemporary term used to describe those surgical interventions the aim of which is to manage disease associated with endodontic and extraradicular apical infection. Disease may present at portals of exit along the length of the root relating to the apical foramen, lateral canals or even iatrogenic perforations. Cases may also involve the periodontium or be concomitant with periodontal lesions. Thus the term "apicectomy", which simply implies removal of the root end, is regarded as an oversimplification for what may be technically challenging surgery involving both periodontal and periapical hard and soft tissues. The term "orthograde" refers to conventional root canal therapy and "retrograde" implies a surgical approach to periapical disease.

In the last five years, significant changes have taken place in technique, armamentarium and materials that render periradicular surgery a more predictable treatment modality. The frequent coexistence of periapical and periodontal infection and the common principles underpinning surgical approaches to managing extraradicular infection require the periodontal surgeon to have knowledge of, and be competent in, periradicular surgery.

Orthograde Retreatment or Periradicular Surgery?

In view of the microbial basis of endodontic disease, treatment efforts (non-surgical or surgical) must aim to eradicate this infection wherever possible. As the infection is most frequently located within the root canal system, orthograde endodontics is normally the most appropriate initial strategy and should always be carried out in the first instance. When infected canals are treated surgically, the root end restoration will simply seal over such infection and predispose to treatment failure through bacterial leakage (Fig 6-1a–c).

Orthograde endodontic instrumentation and irrigation cannot always render canals free from bacteria owing to the anatomic complexity of the root canal system and the resilient nature of microbial biofilms. In some instances, apical biofilms on the external surface of the root and extraradicular infection have been demonstrated (Fig 6-2). These are clearly not amenable to orthograde root canal treatment. A key decision for the periodontist to make, therefore, is whether the existing orthograde root filling can be improved prior to adoption of a surgical approach.

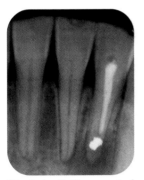 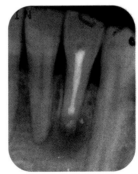 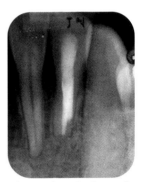

Fig 6-1a Failing surgical endodontic treatment. There is a large periapical radiolucency, an incomplete root resection and an amalgam root-end filling. The root-end filling was not continuous with the root filling.

Fig 6-1b Failing surgical retreatment. A second attempt at periradicular surgery, though technically improved, has failed to resolve the apical pathology.

Fig 6-1c Orthograde retreatment and subsequent healing. Thorough exploration revealed a second untreated canal (common in lower incisors). Respect for basic endodontic principles will provide an environment for predictable healing in most cases.

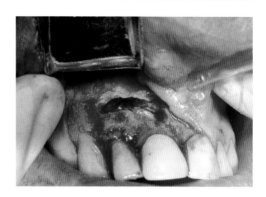

Fig 6-2 A well-organised biofilm is present apically on the external surface of the root of a central incisor. This was independent of any periodontal pocketing.

Case Selection

Indications for Periradicular Surgery
- If orthograde retreatment is not possible.
- Where iatrogenic errors, e.g. perforation, necessitate a surgical approach.
- When retreatment by orthograde approach has failed.
- If extraradicular reasons for failure are suspected:
  – infection
  – cyst
  – foreign body reaction.
- Where cost/patient convenience precludes dismantling of existing restorations.
- When previous surgical endodontics has failed owing to technical inadequacy.

Contraindications for Periradicular Surgery
As with any surgical procedure, there are a few absolute contraindications to periradicular surgery. These have been considered in previous chapters.

Holistic Restorative Treatment Planning
When contemplating periradicular surgery, some general considerations should include:
- stability and prognosis of the remaining dentition
- presence of untreated or unstable periodontal disease
- use of an existing denture to which the tooth may be added, without compromising periodontal health.

A flap with two vertical relieving incisions (Fig 6-6) minimises tissue tension.

A flap design with one relieving incision may provide adequate surgical access where roots are short. This has the advantage of providing easier closure when surgery is complete.

The indications for submarginal flap designs are limited. The use of a semilunar flap is now considered outmoded because access can be poor as it is difficult to predict the size of the lesion from a radiograph. The lesion can therefore extend further than the incision. Where the incision crosses the site of the lesion, this creates a risk of ingress of debris and bacteria to the surgical site, thereby inhibiting healing. As a general principle, flap margins should be replaced on sound bone. In addition, healing of the semilunar flap often results in an unaesthetic raised scar (Fig 6-7).

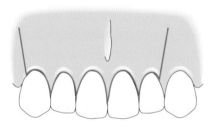 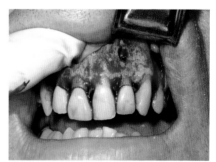

Fig 6-6 Two vertical relieving incisions allow excellent access to single or multiple teeth. In addition this design minimises tissue tension, subsequent operator fatigue and maximises access.

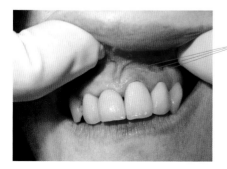

raised semilunar scar

Fig 6-7 An unaesthetic semilunar scar left by failed periradicular surgery. This case required surgical re-treatment.

The Ochsenbein–Luebke flap has been described as a scalloped submarginal incision with vertical relieving incisions (Fig 6-8). This flap is designed to minimise gingival recession and to facilitate comfortable tooth cleaning after surgery. The incision should be made in attached gingivae and not involve the gingival sulcus. Cases therefore should be carefully selected as they require a broad band of attached gingivae. This flap offers more limited access than a marginal incision and is not appropriate where there is periodontal pocketing.

The papilla sparing flap, a hybrid marginal and submarginal flap, has a design that provides good access but minimises papillary recession (Fig 6-9).

Incision
Modern periradicular surgery is best performed using a microsurgical approach. Wherever possible, the use of magnifying loupes provides greater detail of the surgical field. The need for a wide field of vision often limits the

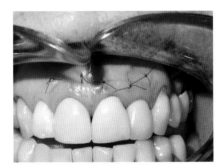

Fig 6-8 Ochsenbein–Luebke flap 48 hours post surgery.

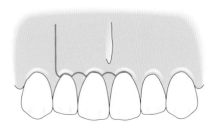

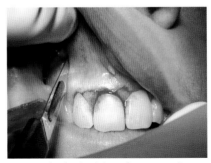

Fig 6-9 The papilla sparing flap involves an intrasulcular incision that spares interdental papillae. These are left in place when the flap is raised (papilla preservation).

use of the operating microscope to root-end management. Microsurgical blades allow for precise anatomic dissection of papillae and round cervical margins. A standard number 15 blade, however, is still invaluable for vertical relieving incisions. Incisions should be down to bone for a full-thickness mucoperiosteal flap.

Vertical relieving incisions should be placed between root eminences; tissue here is thicker and easier to handle, and there is less risk of sloughing and flap necrosis. There may be a dehiscence or fenestration in the bone over the root eminence, particularly around maxillary canines. If flap margins cross these defects, there is an increased risk of post-operative recession.

Reflection
Sharp elevators render raising the flap more predictable and minimise crushing of the marginal tissues. Often where there is a long-standing sinus tract, the flap will be tethered and local sharp dissection may be necessary (Fig 6-10).

Root End Identification and Curettage
Where a large lesion exists, identifying the root end is usually straightforward. A sharp probe can be used to confirm the presence and location of the lesion or to puncture a thin overlying bony plate (Fig 6-11).

Where there has been loss of the buccal bony plate, there is often sufficient access to remove granulation tissue and visualise the root end. Where this is not possible, ostectomy of the buccal plate with a handpiece and burr may be carried out. This should be large enough to allow removal of the lesion

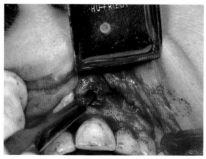

Fig 6-10 Dissecting a tethered flap.

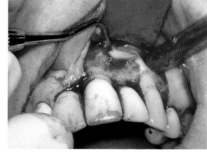

Fig 6-11 A probe confirms the location of the bony lesion.

and examination of the root end. Granulation tissue should be removed from the bony crypt with sharp excavators and curettes. An attempt should be made to remove all granulation tissue because extraradicular infection is a possible reason for failure of the initial treatment. As granulation tissue bleeds readily, full removal will also help to maintain a dry surgical field and thus improve visibility. Removal of granulation tissue should not, however, be at the expense of anatomically sensitive structures.

Root End Resection

The root end of the tooth should usually be resected. It is not possible to render the apical third of root canals free from bacteria in all but the simplest of endodontic cases. In addition, the apical root canal frequently contains deltas, fins and anastamoses where more than one canal is present. It is recommended that 3 mm is removed from the apex for this reason. Where there has been extensive resorption of the apex or the root end has previously been resected, the operator should exercise judgement as further resection may leave a tooth with compromised support. Root-end resection should be carried out with a fluted tungsten carbide fissure burr (Fig 6-12). This leaves the smoothest root end.

It is recommended that the angle of root resection should be carried out as close to perpendicular to the long axis of the root as possible. This will ensure that all accessory canal anatomy is included in the resection (Fig 6-13). A horizontal resection also ensures that minimum dentinal tubules are exposed and thus leakage is reduced (Fig 6-14).

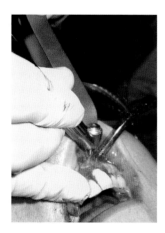

Fig 6-12 A 45° back-venting high-speed surgical turbine with fluted tungsten carbide fissure burr used for root-end resection.

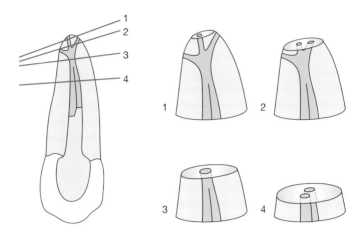

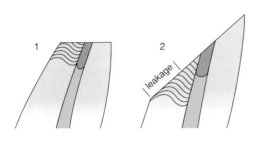

Fig 6-13 A horizontal resection ensures all accessory anatomy is managed with minimal loss of tooth structure.

Fig 6-14 An oblique resection exposes more dentinal tubules and potentiates leakage.

It may be difficult to judge the completeness of root-end resection in some instances. A tactile and visual appreciation of the differences between bone and dentine is helpful here. A methylene blue indicator dye may be used to stain the periodontal ligament round the root (Fig 6-15).

Crypt Control

When the root end has been resected, careful control of the crypt will provide haemostasis and improve visibility and moisture control for root end filling. The use of epinephrine-impregnated cotton wool balls, or "Racellets", applied with pressure at the base of the crypt is useful (Fig 6-16).

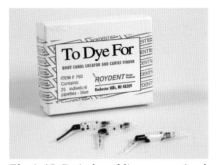

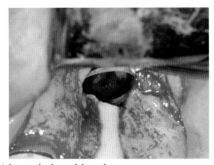

Fig 6-15 Periodontal ligament stained with methylene blue dye.

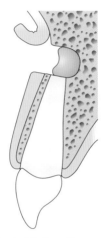

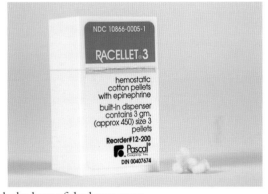

Fig 6-16 Racellets used to pack the base of the bony crypt.

The remainder of the crypt can be packed with Telfa pads, which have the advantage of being fibre-free (Fig 6-17).

When root-end preparation is carried out, the pads can then be removed leaving the Racellet at the base of the crypt to maintain haemostasis. The root end may then be inspected with specially designed "micromirrors" (Fig 6-18). This inspection may reveal a single canal or multiple canals with anastamoses. The root-end preparation should address all accessory anatomy that is present. Often the operating microscope is helpful for detecting and preparing such microanatomy.

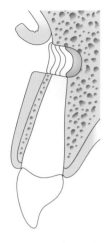

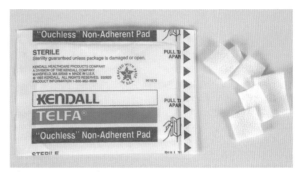

Fig 6-17 Telfa pads aiding haemostasis in the crypt.

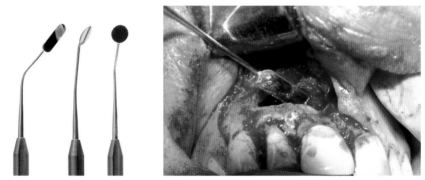

Fig 6-18 Micromirrors and root-end inspection.

Root-end Preparation

Techniques for root-end preparation have changed significantly in recent years. The use of ultrasonic instruments has revolutionised root-end management. Ultrasonic tips have been designed to allow easy access for preparation of the root end in the long axis of the canal. This is not achievable with a traditional handpiece and round burr as the size of the head of the handpiece (even with microheaded handpieces) precludes achieving this angulation (Figs 6-19, 6-20).

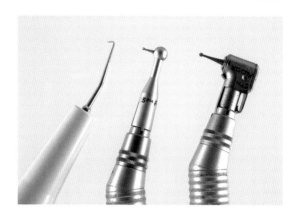

Fig 6-19 Relative sizes of ultrasonic handpiece, microhead handpiece and traditional handpieces.

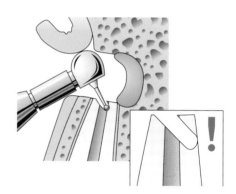

Fig 6-20 The size of traditional hand-pieces renders long axis angulation and root-end preparation difficult. This may lead to inadvertent perforation that is very difficult to detect.

Ultrasonic retropreparation tips are available in a variety of sizes and angulations and are used with a water irrigant for cooling. Diamond-coated tips will rapidly prepare the canal (Fig 6-21), the tip end being 3 mm in length; this is considered the minimum depth for root-end filling in order to minimise leakage.

Ultrasonic preparation will soften the apical gutta percha, which is subsequently removed by aspiration. Any residual apical gutta percha can be plugged coronally with a micropacker (Fig 6-22). The root end may be dried with paper points in preparation for the root-end restoration.

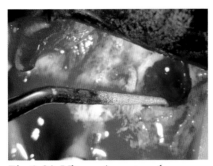

Fig 6-21 Ultrasonic root-end preparation.

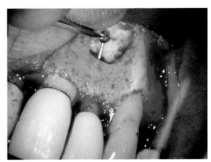

Fig 6-22 Coronal condensation of apical gutta percha.

Root-end Restoration

Many materials have been described for root-end restoration, but the use of amalgam is now outmoded. This material is not tissue-compatible, and breakdown products can cause tattooing (argyria) of oral tissues.

The following materials are recommended for contemporary root-end filling:
- Super EBA (ethoxybenzoic acid)
- IRM (intermediate restorative material)
- MTA (mineral trioxide aggregate)

The former two materials are resin-modified zinc oxide and eugenol cements. These have good handling properties and are useful where access or moisture control is difficult. A fine roll is mixed, and the material is applied with a flat plastic instrument and positioned with a ball-ended burnisher. Again, a micropacker may be useful to condense coronally (Fig 6-23).

MTA is an increasingly popular material in both conventional endodontic treatment and periradicular surgery (Fig 6-24). It is very tissue-compatible and tolerant of moisture; indeed its setting reaction requires the presence of moisture. It is, however, difficult to handle, expensive and technique-sensitive, and is placed with specially designed MTA carriers (Figs 6-25, 6-26).

Orthograde placement of MTA where surgery is planned obviates the need for root-end preparation and filling (Figs 6-27a-c). The material should be at least 6 mm thick to allow for 3 mm of root-end resection and a 3 mm apical barrier.

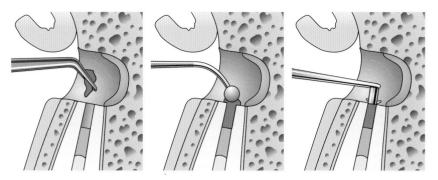

Fig 6-23 IRM or Super EBA placement technique. Retaining the cotton wool pellet at the base of the cavity during preparation and filling will prevent debris falling to the base of the crypt.

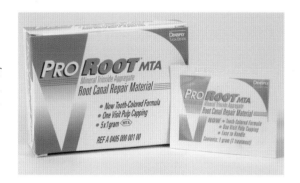

Fig 6-24 Constituents of MTA (75% Portland cement, 20% bismuth oxide, 5% calcium sulphate). Calcium sulphate improves handling characteristics and bismuth sulphate provides radiopacity.

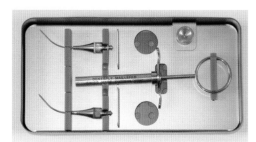

Fig 6-25 MTA carrier.

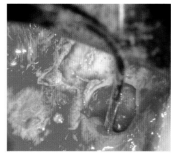

Fig 6-26 MTA placement.

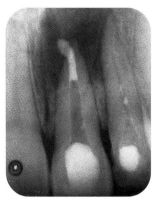
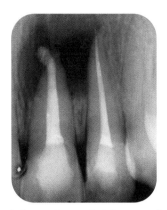

Fig 6-27a Radiograph of non-vital anterior teeth. These teeth had not responded to long-term calcium hydroxide treatment. A 6 mm MTA apical plug was placed in the central incisor and orthograde treatment was carried out on the upper left lateral incisor.

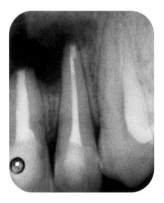

Fig 6-27b These teeth failed to respond to orthograde endodontic treatment and surgery was deemed necessary. The root end of the upper left central incisor was simply resected whereas the tooth UL2 had root-end resection, root-end preparation and retrograde filling with MTA. Note the almost horizontal root resections and characteristic shape of ultrasonic root-end cavity preparation in the upper left lateral incisor.

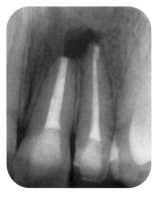

Fig 6-27c Review at 11 months revealed an excellent healing response. It is important to note that cases such as this, with through and through buccopalatal bone loss, will not usually have complete bony infill. This is described as an apical scar and is distinct from a residual periapical lesion.

Closure

When root-end fillings have been placed, the cavity should be debrided carefully of excess root-end filling materials and any cotton pellets removed from the base of the crypt. The cavity should be washed with sterile saline. If MTA has been placed, this should be protected with a flat plastic instrument during irrigation as it sets slowly over 24 hours and may inadvertently be washed out.

A radiograph should ideally be exposed prior to flap closure to assess completeness, angle of root resection and quality of root-end fillings. At this stage these may be revised simply. The flap will normally be closed with fine-diameter synthetic suture materials.

Post-surgical Management

- pain control
- oral hygiene measures
- suture removal
- follow-up.

The mainstays of post-surgical care have been detailed in Chapter 1.

As healing of well-apposed wound edges by primary intention is expected in periradicular surgery, sutures may be removed as early as two days after surgery. Patients should be followed up at six months initially, and then annually thereafter. Radiographic and clinical assessment of healing should be documented at these recall intervals. Radiographic review has been suggested up to four years following surgery, as some cases may be slow to heal.

Modern periradicular surgery provides predictable treatment outcomes where case selection is appropriate and surgical technique is meticulous.

Key Points

- Always consider carefully the quality of the orthograde root filling before considering a surgical approach to therapy.
- Good orthograde endodontics is essential to successful periradicular surgery.
- Consider flap design carefully and account for aesthetic issues and pocketing.

- Ensure base of flap is broader than coronal aspect for good blood supply.
- Repeat incisions where necessary to ensure the delicate elevation of a full-thickness mucoperiosteal flap.
- Ensure vertical relieving incisions are not over "dead space".
- Use a horizontal root-end resection.
- Use ultrasonic root-end preparation.
- Moisture control and haemostasis are essential for root-end visualisation.
- Use an operating microscope or loupes to maximise root-end visualisation.
- Remove 3 mm of apex if possible.
- Use a contemporary restorative material for sealing the root end.

Further Reading

Trope M (ed). Endodontic topics volume 11. Endodontic apical surgery: a delineation of contemporary concepts. Singapore: Blackwell Munksgaard, 2005:1–282.

Chapter 7
Resective Hard Tissue Surgery

Aim

To review the factors influencing the surgical management of molar teeth with furcation involvement and to outline the resective surgical procedures available to facilitate complete and partial tooth retention as an adjunct to restorative care.

Outcome

Having read this chapter the reader should be aware of the various resective treatment approaches available for molar teeth with furcation involvement and/or combined periodontal–endodontic lesions. The reader should understand that the choice of treatment depends upon several interrelated factors.

Introduction

Loss of alveolar bone support arises as a result of inflammatory periodontal disease. Variations in the morphology of multirooted teeth are important in determining at what stage in the periodontal breakdown process a "furcation" area will become involved. A furcation is defined as the point at which the roots of a tooth divide. Furcation lesions involve bone resorption and attachment loss between the roots of multirooted teeth resulting predominantly from periodontal bone loss.

Evidence exists to suggest that molar teeth with furcation involvement have a reduced prognosis. This can be explained partly by the difficulties in obtaining proper access for instrumentation of teeth with complex furcation anatomy, but largely by a patient's inability to effect adequate plaque control, resulting in a persistence of pathogenic microbial flora.

The treatment, management and long-term retention of molar teeth with furcation involvement is challenging. Resective and regenerative techniques have been designed to overcome the difficulties encountered in debridement and maintenance of furcation areas. Regenerative surgery has been discussed in Chapter 5, and therefore this chapter will limit discussion to resective surgical management.

Resective surgery aims to:
1. Establish a favourable anatomy at the dentogingival interface that improves patient access and is conducive to high standards of hygiene.
2. Maintain a healthy and functional tooth with acceptable aesthetics.

Furcation plasty is the reshaping of interradicular bone (osteoplasty) and/or tooth substance (odontoplasty) at the level of the furcation entrance to re-establish soft tissue morphology and allow access for cleaning.

Tunnel preparation is the surgical exposure and management of a furcation area by removal of interradicular bone and apically repositioning of the flaps to facilitate interradicular cleaning. This technique may obviate the need for endodontic treatment and prosthetic reconstruction.

Root amputation is the removal of one whole root of a multirooted tooth, leaving the crown intact. It is appropriate largely for maxillary molars.

Hemisection is the division of a tooth with removal of a root with its accompanying crown portion. This is normally appropriate for mandibular molar teeth. In some cases both halves of the tooth may be retained, leaving two separate roots which are treated as separate teeth.

Examination, diagnosis and treatment planning

Hard tissue resective therapy is a technically demanding procedure that relies upon careful case selection and interdisciplinary treatment planning to optimise success. Treatment usually includes endodontic therapy, periodontal surgery and prosthodontic reconstruction. Consideration must be given to factors such as tooth restorability, occlusal factors and the strategic value of the tooth prior to embarking upon treatment.

Improved endodontic management and the increased sophistication of periodontal surgery provide the means to consider retaining molar teeth with furcation problems that would otherwise have been lost.

The unique, complex anatomy of the root favours the development of periodontitis and bone loss in the furcation area. Important anatomical features of the furcation area include:

- the size of the root furcation
- root concavities
- cervical enamel projections
- bifurcation ridges
- enamel pearls.

These features hamper access for routine periodontal debridement. Loss of vitality may arise because of the presence of accessory canals in the furcation area. These provide pathways that allow passage of bacteria between the pulp and periodontium, thereby creating a concomitant periodontal-endodontic lesion.

Studies that have assessed the response of teeth with furcation involvement to traditional surgical and non-surgical therapy have all reported decreased success rates compared with teeth without furcal disease.

Furcation involvement can be classified (Hamp's Classification, 1975) according to the amount of periodontal bone loss that has occurred in the interradicular area (Fig 7-1).

Grade I: Horizontal loss of periodontal support not exceeding one third of the width of the tooth.
Grade II: Horizontal loss of periodontal support exceeding one third of the width of the tooth, but not encompassing the total width of the furcation area.
Grade III: Horizontal "through and through" destruction of the periodontal tissues in the furcation area.

The extent and the severity of periodontal bone loss is assessed by a combination of clinical and radiographic examinations. Radiographic examination should consist of periapical radiographs taken using a paralleling technique to allow comprehensive endodontic assessment and analysis of bone levels. The use of a conventional periodontal probe will allow

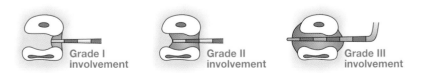

Fig 7-1 Hamp's Classification of a furcation.

assessment of probing pocket depth and clinical attachment loss, which are measured in a vertical dimension, but will not allow negotiation and exploration of the three-dimensional aspect of the furcation area. The presence and depth of furcations may be examined with a specific, curved furcation probe (Fig 7-2). The examination of interproximal furcations in maxillary molars and premolars can be difficult owing to problems of access.

For the majority of teeth, a conventional non-surgical approach including RSD should be employed in the first instance. If this approach is unsuccessful or inappropriate, consideration can be given to other treatment options (Box 7-1), which include resective procedures.

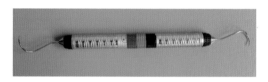

Fig 7-2   A furcation probe (Nabers probe, Hu–Friedy).

Box 7-1 **Treatment options for molar teeth with furcation involvement**

- Scaling and RSD
- Surgical RSD
- Furcation plasty
- Tunnelling procedures
- Root amputation
- Hemisection
- Regeneration procedures
- Apically repositioned flap
- Extraction and prosthetic replacement
- Implant placement

Indications for Root Amputation/Resection and Hemisection
- Advanced periodontal bone loss affecting one root.
- Grade II and Grade III furcation involvement.
- Complex anatomy impeding oral hygiene, which would be facilitated by removal of a root.
- Failing endodontic treatment in one root that is not amenable to retreatment or periradicular surgery. Periradicular surgery may be more difficult to perform on a posterior tooth than an anterior tooth. For this reason,

the relatively simpler techniques of root amputation or hemisection may be considered.

- Severe recession or dehiscence of bone covering a root.
- Bone loss around a periodontal–endodontic lesion that is compromising bone support for an adjacent sound root, or an adjacent tooth (Fig 7-3).
- Root fracture.
- Difficult access to caries within a furcation.
- External root resorption or root caries affecting one root.

Fig 7-3a Radiolucency and bone loss around distal root of first molar.

Fig 7-3b Root canal and periodontal treatment did not resolve the intrabony pathology and the bone level mesial to the LR7 was compromised.

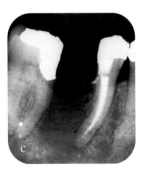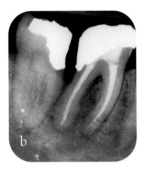

Fig 7-3c Six months following hemisection, note the restoration of bone mesial to the lower right second permanent molar.

Fig 7-3d Temporary crown, lab-made to facilitate plaque control.

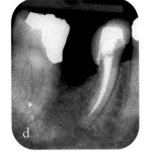

Fig 7-3e Definitive crown, made elsewhere. It is worth noting that the definitive crown has a poor design and emergence profile, compared to the temporary crown. The definitive crown had to be remade to facilitate longer-term maintenance of plaque control.

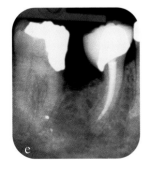

Contraindications to Resective Surgery
• Poor oral hygiene.
• Unwillingness of patient to undergo complex restorative and surgical treatment.
• Poor long-term prognosis.
• Poorly executed endodontic treatment in all roots.
• Any medical condition that contraindicates surgery.

Assessment of Teeth for Resective Surgery

Tooth-specific Assessment
• Endodontic assessment including the quality of pre-existing endodontic treatment.
• The anatomy of the roots. Sufficient separation of the roots is required so that resection is possible without damaging adjacent roots. It is important to ensure that there will be enough bone remaining around the roots that are to be retained. Fused or closely approximated roots are not suitable candidates for resection. This point is illustrated in Fig 7-4.
• Adequate access for surgery.
• The location of the disease will usually determine which root is to be retained or removed. In some circumstances the final decision as to which roots are to be retained is left until the time of surgery. Direct visual access to the root anatomy at this time allows better assessment.

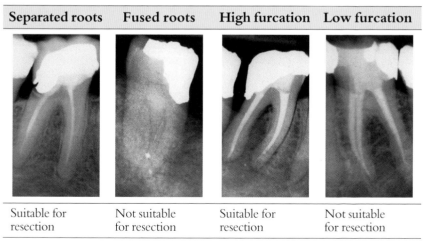

Separated roots	Fused roots	High furcation	Low furcation
Suitable for resection	Not suitable for resection	Suitable for resection	Not suitable for resection

Fig 7-4 Furcation anatomy and its suitability for resective surgery.

- Restorability of the remaining root.
- Diminutive roots may exhibit mobility following resection of the other root. The remainder of the periodontal attachment apparatus around the remaining root(s) and their anticipated stability must be carefully considered by assessing crown/root ratios and also residual bone support.
- Aesthetic considerations following resection.

General Assessment
- Medical history.
- Oral hygiene.
- Periodontal and restorative status of remaining dentition.
- Financial commitment.
- Time commitment.
- The operator's experience and skill.

Some additional tooth-specific considerations are listed in Box 7-2.

Box 7-2 **Tooth specific considerations in planning – root anatomy**

- The distal-buccal root of the maxillary first molar and the distal root of the mandibular first molar have the smallest root surface areas, and if all other factors are equal these roots are preferentially resected.

- The superimposition of the palatal root on a radiograph film may conceal the actual bony morphology in the interradicular area in maxillary molars.

- The average furcation entrance diameter is smaller than the tips of conventional hand instruments.

- In mandibular molars, endodontic treatment is generally more straightforward in distal roots. Furthermore, mesial roots often have a concavity on their distal aspect, which makes oral hygiene more difficult.

- Mandibular first molars may have a second distal root.

- The mesiobuccal root of maxillary first molars has two canals in over 90% of cases and can be difficult to treat endodontically. This root often has a broad flat shape buccopalatally and resection may be challenging.

Procedure

Presurgical Preparation

Informed consent for resective hard tissue surgery needs to include a balanced discussion of risks and benefits along with other treatment options and their predictability. A review of the literature relating to root resection shows there is no consensus regarding the success rates of such procedures. Studies have examined different procedures and measured different outcomes, thus making inter-study comparisons and the drawing of conclusions complex. Several studies have evaluated the long-term effectiveness of root resection procedures and have shown significant variations in success rates of between 62% and 100%. Failure of treatment can be periodontal in nature; however, endodontic complications and root fractures frequently contribute to failure and this must be discussed with the patient. Box 7-3 lists some of the potential complications that can arise following treatment.

Box 7-3 **Potential complications following treatment**

- Pain and swelling.
- Reshaped root surface being more susceptible to caries.
- Root fracture.
- Root sensitivity (tunnel procedure or furcation plasty).
- Failure of endodontic therapy.
- Continued periodontal destruction.
- Failure of treatment owing to trauma from occlusion.

The following must all be carried out prior to surgery:
- Treatment planning for endodontic treatment.
- Construction of a provisional restoration.
- Planning for tooth preparation during surgery.
- Planning of the final prosthetic reconstruction.

Patients must be aware of the degree of time and financial commitment that such procedures may necessitate.

When should endodontic treatment be performed?

As a general rule, endodontic treatment should be carried out prior to resective therapy. In some cases the need for resection is only identified whilst carrying out periodontal surgery. In these emergency situations, resection should be carried out and endodontic treatment initiated as soon as possible after resection to avoid complications such as pulpitis and internal crown/root resorption. Following resection of a vital root, the crown should be sealed with a suitable restorative material.

For elective resection procedures, a suitable core buildup restoration is required following endodontic treatment and prior to resection, ensuring that it is retentive in each individual root. The core buildup should also provide appropriate retention and resistance for the subsequent full coverage restoration. The use of posts should be avoided, if possible, as evidence suggests these may predispose to root fracture.

Furcation Plasty

This is, in the main, an outmoded procedure which involves the reshaping of the alveolar bone and root dentine to produce a contour that is conducive to home care. This technique should be used judiciously as it carries the risk of pulp exposure, dentinal hypersensitivity and caries. It is rarely performed owing to the availability of more conservative treatment options aimed at tissue regeneration.

Tunnelling

Tunnelling is the intentional creation of a Class III furcation defect by interradicular bone recontouring to make the furcation entrance accessible for cleaning with a mini-interdental brush. This procedure is only suitable when the furcation entrance is wide and coronally positioned to allow for easy passage of the interdental brush. The use of this technique is reserved mainly for mandibular first molars.

The surgical procedure involves intrasulcular incision and retraction of a full-thickness mucoperiosteal envelope flap, buccally and lingually. The furcation area requires thorough debridement to remove granulation tissue and hard tissue deposits such as calculus. Odontoplasty and osteoplasty can be carried out using ultrasonics, hand or rotary instruments, or a combination of these. The intrafurcal bone is removed in a vertical direction; it is also necessary to reduce the alveolar bone around the roots next to the furcation to a level slightly apical to the level of the intra-furcal bone. This is to prevent gingival rebound closing up the furcation entrance. Alternatively, a plastic wedge secured by dental floss may be inserted into the opened furcation, prior to flap closure. If covered by a surgical dressing and left for two weeks, re-epithelialisation arises apically to the furcation and retains patency. Following the creation of a "tunnel", the soft tissues are apically repositioned to expose the furcation.

Factors favourable to a successful outcome for a tunnelling procedure include:
- Mandibular molars.
- Long roots.
- High furcation entrance.
- Widely separated roots.
- For vital teeth, the floor of the pulp chamber should not be close to the roof of the furcation to avoid perforation.
- The patient should be at low risk of developing caries.

Root Amputation and Hemisection

The basic principles of contemporary periodontal surgery discussed in Chapter 1 apply to these procedures.

The surgical procedure utilises an intrasulcular incision followed by retraction of a full-thickness mucoperiosteal envelope flap to expose the furcation area. In some cases, where the furcation area is already exposed, roots can be amputated without raising a flap. Having achieved adequate exposure of the furcation, root amputation or hemisection is carried out using a fine diamond burr in a back-venting air rotor (to prevent surgical emphysema). It is often practical to section the supragingival hard tissue prior to elevating the surgical flap, using an air rotor. If this approach is undertaken, it is vital to locate the furcation using a probe and to direct the burr cut towards this area, with the location probe *in situ* as a direction guide.

For a hemisection (Fig 7–5a–h), the burr is held parallel to the tooth axis and the tooth is sectioned from the buccal aspect towards the lingual aspect. A small elevator can be inserted at this stage and twisted slightly to assess

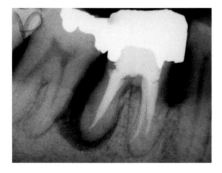

Fig 7–5a Radiograph of a lower right first permanent molar, which required hemisection. Owing to acute symptoms it was necessary to section the tooth before placement of an amalgam core restoration to fill and seal the pulp chamber, prior to surgical sectioning. Ideally, the pulp chamber should be filled with amalgam prior to hemisection to provide a good seal at the time of surgery and prevent ingress of bacteria.

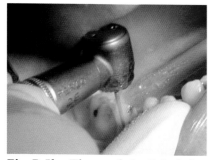

Fig 7-5b The tooth in 7-5a being sectioned using an air rotor and tapered fine fissure diamond burr, prior to raising the surgical flap.

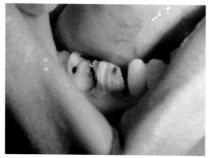

Fig 7-5c The tooth in 7-5b with the buccal cut completed.

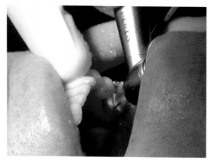

Fig 7-5d The tooth in 7-5c at the time of lingual sectioning.

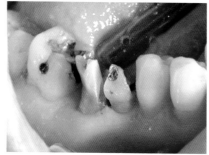

Fig 7-5e The tooth in 7-5d sectioned completely.

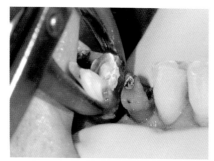

Fig 7-5f Removal of the distal half of the tooth using forceps (normally elevators are used).

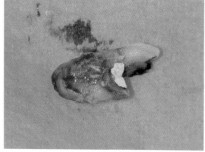

Fig 7-5g The removed half of the tooth.

119

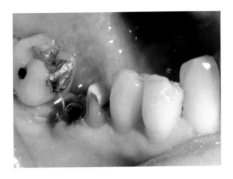

Fig 7-5h The retained half sealed coronally with glass ionomer core material.

whether sectioning is complete. When separation is confirmed the root is gently elevated, avoiding pressure on the root to be retained.

For root amputation, the root is sectioned horizontally using a fine diamond burr at the base of the crown and the sectioned root gently elevated (Fig 7-6).

Care is required to avoid damaging the adjacent roots and periodontal tissues. Following root amputation or hemisection, the socket is debrided to remove granulation tissue and the bony defect that remains around the residual root may be recontoured to produce a form that facilitates plaque control. The

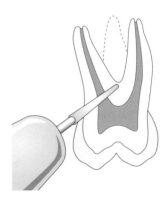

Fig 7-6 Burr position for root resection.

remaining root or roots are then visualised and probed and any remaining hard tissue projections smoothed with a fine diamond burr. Where any tooth preparation or temporary crown cementation is performed after root elevation, the socket should be packed with gauze to help prevent entry of debris into the socket. Before final closure, the pack should be removed and final irrigation carried out.

In rare cases where resection has been carried out prior to endodontic treatment, the crown should be sealed with a suitable restorative material at the time of surgery. Flap closure is performed with simple interrupted sutures; in some cases (maxillary molar root amputation) it may be necessary to reposition the flap apically to expose the furcation.

Some teeth may require a provisional full coverage restoration directly after resection. Care must be taken to remove excess cement following cementation of the restoration.

Definitive Restoration
Tooth resection procedures should be designed to preserve as much tooth structure as practical. Several factors need to be considered when restoring root resected molar teeth because of the unique residual anatomy following resection.

Factors to be considered include:
• type of resection
• existing restorative status
• periodontal status
• occlusion.

The root surface may require recontouring to remove the root stump or overhanging dentine spicules. Incomplete removal of residual ledges creates plaque-retentive factors that may aggravate or potentiate periodontal problems (Fig 7-7).

Consideration must be given to achieving adequate retention and resistance form for crown preparation of a resected tooth. When providing a crown restoration, a favourable emergence profile from the preparation margin is essential for establishing an environment where plaque control is more easily maintained.

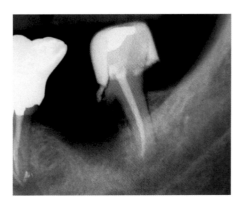

Fig 7-7 Incomplete removal of furcation.

During crown preparation it is important not to reduce excessively the dentinal walls as this may lead to increased risk of root fracture, and often a chamfer preparation is most appropriate. Supragingival crown margins are more favourable than subgingival margins to facilitate maintenance of good plaque control.

It has been demonstrated that occlusal forces exacerbate the bone loss caused by periodontitis. It is therefore important to assess the risk of occlusal trauma and make occlusal alterations as necessary. Crown design should include the prescription of a narrow occlusal table and shallow cuspal inclines to reduce occlusal loading. The occlusal scheme should avoid significant guidance. The photographic sequence (Fig 7-8a–e) illustrates the hemisection of two mandibular molars with crown restoration.

The photographic sequence (Fig 7-9a–f) illustrates the hemisection of two mandibular molars, both of which had unrestorable root caries, followed by placement of copings and a metal–ceramic bridge.

The photographic sequence (Fig 7-10a–d) illustrates the endodontic treatment and root amputation of the distobuccal root of a maxillary molar.

Following restoration, the patient will require specific oral hygiene advice to maintain a plaque-free environment (Fig 7-11).

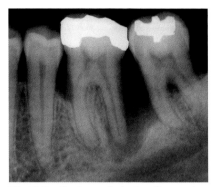

Fig 7-8a Perio-endo lesion first molar, furcation lesion second molar.

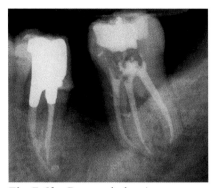

Fig 7-8b Post endodontic treatment and hemisection of first molar.

Fig 7-8c Radiograph showing crown restorations.

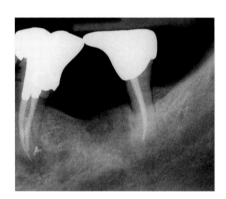

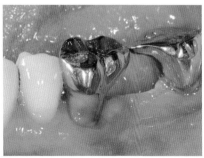

Fig 7-8d Buccal view of crowns, note ease of access to cleansing.

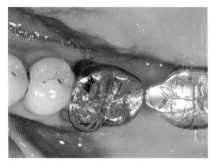

Fig 7-8e Occlusal view of crowns, note small occlusal table.

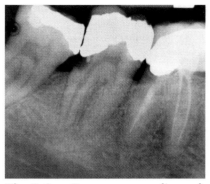

Fig 7-9a Pretreatment radiograph showing poor root filling (first molar) and caries (second molar).

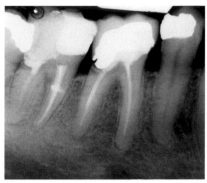

Fig 7-9b Post-endodontic retreatment.

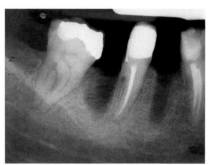

Fig 7-9c Radiograph shows hemisection of two molars.

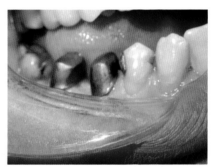

Fig 7-9d Gold copings on hemisected teeth.

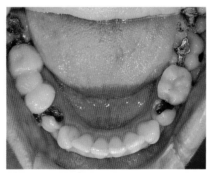

Fig 7-9e Bridge restoration.

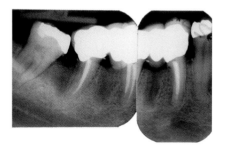

Fig 7-9f Radiograph post bridge placement.

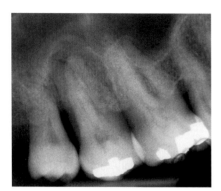

Fig 7-10a Perio-endo lesion.

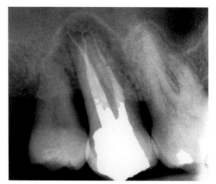

Fig 7-10b Root canal treatment: note core extending into root canal system.

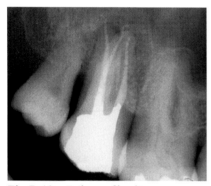

Fig 7-10c Failure of healing.

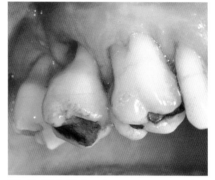

Fig 7-10d Following root amputation distobuccal root.

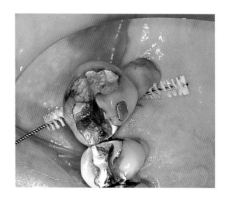

Fig 7-11 Cleansing of the furcation.

Maintenance

Radiographic examination is usually carried out immediately following resection, then at intervals of six months and 12 months. Regular periodontal assessment and maintenance is crucial to the success of the treatment. Maintenance therapy includes periodontal and endodontic evaluation, radiographic review, removal of supragingival and subgingival plaque and calculus deposits, RSD and, importantly, review of the patient's oral hygiene.

Most patients with a history of periodontitis initially require a three-monthly recall programme. Following a satisfactory response to treatment, recall visit intervals can be modified according to individual patient needs. It is important to remember that careful design features incorporated into the definitive extracoronal restoration of resected teeth will greatly facilitate the surgical procedure and improve the prognosis for the tooth (Fig 7-12).

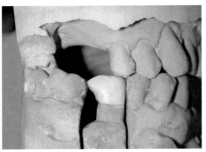

Fig 7-12a A temporary crown constructed in the laboratory to facilitate interproximal plaque control and with a reduced occlusal table to reduce occlusal forces.

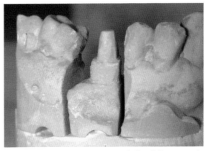

Fig 7-12b A stone model of the tooth in 7-12a prepared for a definitive crown.

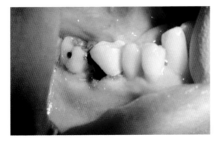

Fig 7-12c The definitive crown for the tooth in 7-12a, with a reduced occlusal table, a contact area with the lower right second permanent molar and easy marginal cleansing.

Key Points

- The treatment of furcations can be a difficult task, which is complicated by variations in local anatomy.
- Success is largely dependent upon careful case selection and selection of teeth that are suitable for resective procedures.
- Another important factor that is necessary for the success of treatment is the patient's ability to maintain good plaque control.
- Resective surgery may involve a considerable amount of treatment on one tooth. It is important that both dentist and patient agree upon the strategic importance of retaining the tooth prior to embarking upon financially demanding and time-consuming treatment.

Further Reading

Al-Shammari KF, Kazor CE, Wang HL. Molar root anatomy and management of furcation defects. J Clin Periodontol 2001;28:730–740.

Carnevale G, Pontoriero R, Hürzeler M. Management of furcation involvement. Periodontol 2000, 1995;9:69–89.

Cattabriga M, Pedrazzoli V, Wilson TG Jr. The conservative approach in the treatment of furcation lesions. Periodontol 2000, 2000;22:133–153.

DeSanctis M, Murphy KG. The role of resective periodontal surgery in the treatment of furcation defects. Periodontol 2000, 2000;22:154–168.

Chapter 8
Crown-lengthening Surgery

Aim

This chapter aims to describe where crown-lengthening surgery is an appropriate adjunct to restorative dental care. The techniques employed in crown-lengthening will be discussed in detail.

Outcome

The reader should understand the principles of, and indications for, crown-lengthening surgery and where it may form a useful adjunct to restorative care. The practical aspects of crown-lengthening described will allow the practitioner to manage simple cases in a predictable manner.

Introduction

Modern restorative dentistry emphasises the holistic management of the patient and the intimate relationship between its three sub-specialties; endodontics, periodontics and fixed and removable prosthetics. Above all, the periodontium forms the foundation for teeth and their restoration and should be the first consideration in any restorative treatment plan. Patients are becoming increasingly aware that gingival aesthetics may be as important as those of the dental hard tissues.

Periodontal surgery is not wholly concerned with managing chronic pathology. The use of periodontal pre-prosthetic surgery may greatly enhance the success of restorations in terms of both retention and also aesthetics. Whilst implant treatment has rendered some more traditional forms of pre-prosthetic surgery obsolete, crown-lengthening surgery is still an indispensable treatment-planning option for the restorative dentist. It is particularly valuable in the treatment of tooth wear, where it can make the difference between a patient becoming a denture wearer and being successfully restored with fixed prostheses. This chapter will therefore focus on case selection and techniques for crown-lengthening.

Tooth-specific assessment
- Local periodontal health.
- Quality of existing restorations.
- Presence of caries.
- Predicted crown: root ratio.
- Proximity of furcations.

Gingival assessment
- Tissue biotype (thick/thin).
- Width of attached gingiva.

Aesthetic considerations
- Surgery in the aesthetic zone.
- Preservation of interdental papillae.
- Impact of crown-lengthening on gingival aesthetics of adjacent teeth.

Alternative treatment options and their predictability
- Orthodontic extrusion of teeth +/- crown-lengthening.
- Overdenture in cases of extreme tooth wear.
- Extraction and tooth replacement.

Presurgical Preparation

General aspects of presurgical preparation have been discussed in Chapter 1.

The following factors are pertinent to crown-lengthening surgery:
- tooth preparation
- informed consent for surgery.

Tooth Preparation
Where possible, the provisional restoration of teeth that are planned for crown-lengthening will simplify further management. Caries should be removed as far as possible initially. This will allow an assessment of the remaining tooth substance and restorability. Existing crown restorations should be removed and replaced with provisional restorations. Provisional crowns can provide a clear guide to the surgeon of encroachment on biological width and where bone removal may be a necessary adjunct to crown-lengthening (Fig 8-2).

In addition, well-fitting margins simplify oral hygiene, reduce plaque accumulation and improve healing responses post-surgery.

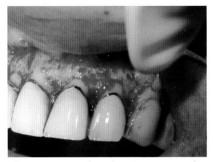

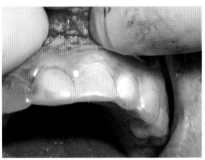

Fig 8-2 Crown-lengthening surgery after placement of gold/composite provisional crowns. Deep margins encroaching on biological width necessitate bone removal in this case.

Fig 8-3 A stent constructed on a diagnostic wax-up, used during crown-lengthening. Alveolar bony crest is visible through the clear stent and may be compared with the planned position of the restoration margins.

In many cases, crown-lengthening is necessary before teeth can be restored, for example in severe tooth surface loss. In such cases preparation of a preoperative diagnostic wax-up is an invaluable planning aid. This will provide information such as how much tooth substance needs to be exposed for crown retention, likely post-operative crown–root ratio and planned aesthetic result. In addition, a stent constructed on the diagnostic wax-up may also be used as a surgical guide for bone removal (Fig 8-3).

Definitive endodontic treatment should be carried out prior to crown-lengthening where appropriate. Failed attempts at root canal treatment after crown-lengthening surgery may result in tooth loss and therefore the patient may have been exposed to unnecessary surgery. Where isolation due to short crown height is difficult, a split dam technique may be used. A case in which a carious tooth was endodontically treated and had subsequent crown-lengthening surgery and post placement over a single visit is illustrated in Fig 8-4 a–e).

Informed Consent
Crown-lengthening surgery has similar risks to other forms of periodontal surgery. In particular, the risk of an adverse aesthetic impact should be discussed carefully. Often this surgery is in the aesthetic zone. Loss of interdental papillae and subsequent "black triangles" may be a significant consequence. Bone removal around teeth adjacent to those to be crown-

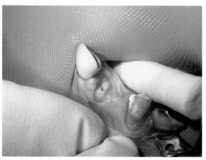

Fig 8-4a After excavation of caries on the incisor bridge abutment, little or no tooth substance is left supragingivally. Note the split rubber dam.

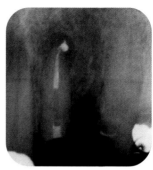

Fig 8-4b Root canal treatment is performed on the tooth and a temporary seal is placed in the access cavity.

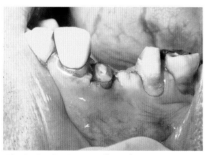

Fig 8-4c An inverse bevel gingivectomy is carried out to lengthen the clinical crown. Two sutures are placed inter-dentally.

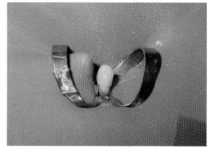

Fig 8-4d The tooth is isolated again and a fibre-based post and composite core are constructed.

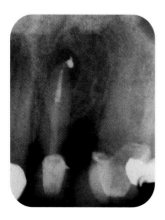

Fig 8-4e The fibre-based post *in situ* and a temporary bridge restoration has been fabricated.

lengthened may compromise their own support. The risk of exposing a furcation has to be carefully evaluated. Exposure of root dentine may also predispose to dentinal hypersensitivity. Orthodontic extrusion of teeth may be valuable in some instances as the alveolar bone and gingivae will tend to move with the tooth. This may help place the gingival margin in an ideal position and prevent excessively long clinical crowns.

Another not uncommon consequence is relapse of the gingival margin (Pontoriero and Carnevale, 2001). Bone removal does not come naturally to periodontists, and where this is inadequate the gingival margin will tend to return to preoperative levels. The surgeon should therefore make every effort to ensure that, where necessary, bone removal is carried out to allow at least 3 mm between alveolar crest and restorative margins. Needless to say, careful clinical records should be made as part of the planning process, and where aesthetic change is intended clinical photographs are mandatory. It may be helpful for the inexperienced operator to construct a diagnostic model with a soft tissue mask so that surgery can be rehearsed (Fig 8-5). It is also important to record a detailed pocket chart around the teeth planned for surgery, to ensure:
1. No untreated periodontitis remains undetected at the planning stage.
2. A detailed record of probing sulcus depth is available at the time of surgery.

Surgical Procedures

There are three main approaches to surgical crown-lengthening:
- gingivectomy
- apically repositioned flap (APF) surgery
- APF with osseous reduction (osteoplasty/ostectomy).

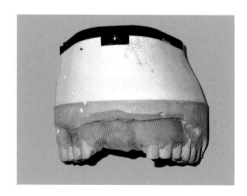

Fig 8-5 A soft tissue mask may be used to rehearse surgery on a model.

135

As bone removal is often necessary to avoid encroaching on biological width, the APF with osseous reduction is probably the most frequently used approach. Each approach, however, will be considered in turn.

Gingivectomy

Gingivectomy represents the simplest approach to crown-lengthening. This has been considered in greater detail in Chapter 3. It is generally appropriate where there is an element of gingival overgrowth or false pocketing. It is also useful where there has been loss of periodontal attachment. In this respect, a detailed pocket chart will be invaluable.

There are two main approaches to gingivectomy for crown-lengthening:
* external bevel incision
* inverse bevel incision.

The inverse bevel incision (as utilised in the modified Widman flap) tends to be more popular than an external bevel incision in this context. This flap design is detailed in Chapter 4.

Precise changes in gingival margin location are relatively straightforward with a gingivectomy technique. This is in contrast to the apically repositioned flap where location of gingival margin may be less predictable and technically more demanding. However, the gingivectomy approach may be less conservative of attached gingival tissue. Where this is only present as a thin band, an APF may represent a more tissue-conservative option.

Apically Repositioned Flap Surgery

Commonly, an inverse bevel incision is initially made for this type of flap. The width of attached gingivae should be carefully assessed, and where this is minimal the incision may be intrasulcular to preserve attached gingiva. Where there is abundant attached gingivae, the incision may be relatively scalloped and parasulcular. Local gingival conditions should be observed, and the flap may incorporate both intrasulcular and parasulcular incisions simultaneously (see Chapter 4).

The flap design for an apically repositioned flap should normally involve two vertical relieving incisions. This increases flap mobility and makes apical repositioning more straightforward. The flap will normally extend to include adjacent teeth and thus allow interdental bone removal and recontouring as appropriate. Often the decision to remove bone can be made when the flap is raised, and precise measurements may be made of the distance between alveolar crest and restoration margins. The relieving incisions should be made as vertical as possible and parallel with each other. This means that when the flap is repositioned apically there is good apposition of flap margins at these relieving incisions.

A case in which an apically repositioned flap was used to lengthen the clinical crowns of two central incisor teeth is illustrated in Fig 8-6.

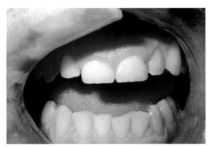

Fig 8-6a The central incisors were crowned after childhood trauma. Impingement on biological width led to gingivitis around these teeth which failed to respond to local oral hygiene measures. The gingival margins of the central incisor teeth are significantly more coronal than the adjacent lateral incisors.

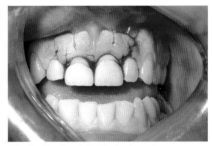

Fig 8-6b An APF is designed to expose the restoration margins and create a harmonious gingival appearance with adjacent lateral incisors. Note the sutures in the labial sulcus. These have the function of shortening the flap and maintaining apical tension during healing.

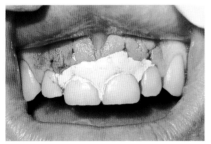

Fig 8-6c A periodontal dressing is placed to help maintain the new apical position of the gingival margin while healing progresses.

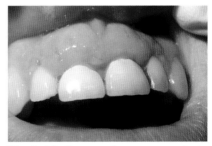

Fig 8-6d One week post-operatively the gingival margins of the restorations are still exposed; however, some relapse of gingival margin is already evident. Greater bone removal during surgery would have created a more stable apical gingival position.

137

When the APF is sutured, it is convenient initially to place sutures in the vertical relieving incisions. The needle penetration in the flap margin should be relatively more apical in the bound tissue than in the reflected flap as this will generate apical rather than coronal tension (Fig 8-7).

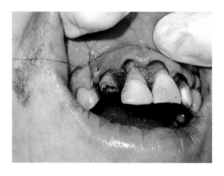

Fig 8-7 Suture positioning in the APF. Needle entry is more apical in bound mucosa than in the reflected flap.

Interdental sutures are placed to provide soft tissue coverage of interdental bone. This is done with minimal tension to avoid coronal movement of the flap. It is very difficult to attain perfect closure of an apically repositioned flap, and in some places healing will be by secondary intention. It is often prudent to place a periodontal dressing after closure to protect any areas of denuded bone.

Osseous Reduction

Osseous reduction during crown-lengthening is frequently necessary. A decision can be made when the flap is raised and measurement of alveolar crest to restoration margin can be made with a periodontal probe. Details on principles of bone removal may be found in Chapter 2. Initial bone removal is accomplished with burrs and copious coolant. An osseous contour is created to mirror the parabolic interdental contour and scalloped cervical margins of the original alveolar bone ideally to support the gingival tissues.

It is important to avoid damage to root surfaces of the teeth to be lengthened. To this end a thin layer of bone is left on the root surfaces. This may then be removed with hand instruments. The Wedelstadt chisel (Fig 8-8a) or Sugarman file (Fig 8-8b) are ideal for this. A sharp curette may also be useful.

Fig 8-8 Precise bone removal with (a) Wedelstadt chisel (b) Sugarman file. (Courtesy of Sato, *Periodontal Surgery: A Clinical Atlas*, 2000)

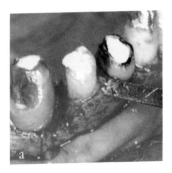
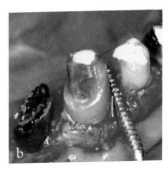

The tissues are then closed as detailed for the APF.

The results obtained following crown-lengthening surgery using the inverse bevel flap (modified Widman flap) can be comparable with the APF (Fig 8-9a,b) but there is less flexibility in repositioning the gingival margin using this approach.

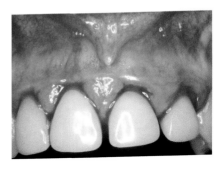

Fig 8-9a Inflamed marginal gingivae following placement of temporary crown restorations with poor subgingival margins, owing to encroachment on the biological width.

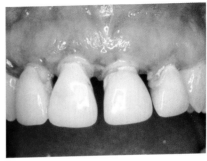

Fig 8-9b The same patient as in Fig 8-9a ten days following an inverse bevel flap and bone removal to render preparation margins supragingival. The poor margins of the temporary crowns can be visualised along with the excess cement lute. Laboratory-made close-fitting temporary crowns should be provided at this stage, prior to allowing the gingival margin to stabilise and fabrication of definitive crowns.

Post-surgical Management

Healing is by secondary intention in many cases, and periodontal dressings and sutures are left in place for about one week where possible. Gingival maturation will continue over time, and it is sensible to postpone definitive restoration of teeth until this time. In particular, definitive restoration of teeth in the aesthetic zone should be carried out at least six months after surgery.

Key Points

- Understand the principle of "biological width" and the role it plays in the need for crown-lengthening and the surgical techniques used therein.
- Carefully consider the aesthetic and dental health impact that crown-lengthening surgery may have.
- Provide high-quality provisional restorations where possible before carrying out surgery.
- Consider the apically repositioned flap with osseous reduction as the technique of first choice for crown-lengthening.
- Postpone definitive restorations until gingival tissue healing is complete.

References

Gargiulo AW, Wentz FM, Orban B. Dimensions and relations of the dentogingival junction in humans. J Periodontol 1961;32:261–267.

Ingber JS, Rose LF, Coslet JG. The "biologic width" – a concept in periodontics and restorative dentistry. Alpha Omegan 1977;70(3):62–65.

Nevins M, Skurow HM. The intracrevicular restorative margin, the biological width and the maintenance of the gingival margin. Int J Periodontics Restorative Dent 1984;3:31–49.

Pontoriero R, Carnevale G. Surgical crown lengthening: a 12-month clinical wound healing study. J Periodontol 2001;72:841–848.

Further Reading

Goodacre CJ, Campagni WV, Aquilino SA. Tooth preparations for complete crowns: an art form based on scientific principles. J Prosthet Dent 2001;85:363–376.

Padbury A Jr, Eber R, Wang HL. Interactions between the gingiva and the margin of restorations. J Clin Periodontol 2003;30:379–385.

Chapter 9
Mucogingival Grafting Procedures
– An Overview

Aim

This chapter aims to describe the different surgical techniques available for managing localised gingival recession. The principal causes of localised gingival recession have been discussed in a previous book in this series (*Periodontal Medicine – A Window on the Body*).

Outcome

At the end of this chapter the reader should be familiar with the different surgical treatment options to augment the gingivae and cover the exposed root when localised recession defects are present. The reader should appreciate that mucogingival surgery can be technically challenging, recognise that there may be limitations to what can be achieved surgically and be able to identify those patients who would be better managed in a specialist care setting.

Introduction

Gingival recession is the exposure of the root surface owing to the apical migration of the gingival margin. Mucogingival therapy (also referred to as periodontal plastic surgery) may be required to:

- prevent further recession
- correct aesthetic problems
- aid plaque control
- reduce dentine hypersensitivity
- prepare a solid tissue bed for implant surgery.

There are several different mucogingival treatment approaches, which usually involve the manipulation of the patient's tissues to augment the gingivae and cover the exposed root.

The latest Adult Dental Health Survey carried out in the UK revealed that 66% of dentate adults had at least one tooth with a root surface that was exposed, worn, filled or decayed. Gingival recession is a common feature in populations with good as well as poor standards of hygiene. It may be localised or generalised in nature.

Risk Factors for Gingival Recession

- **Trauma** – most commonly caused by aggressive tooth-brushing and less commonly factitious injury. This usually results in a localised recession defect.
- **Anatomic factors** – narrow apicocoronal height and decreased buccolingual thickness of the attached gingivae can predispose to gingival recession. This recession usually arises on the buccal surfaces of teeth. Short vestibular depths and prominent fraenal attachments may limit plaque control and therefore potentiate recession.
- **Malaligned teeth** – fenestrations and dehiscences (Fig 9-1a,b) are commonly found around malaligned teeth. These make teeth more susceptible to gingival recession.
- **Postorthodontic therapy** – where labial bodily movement of teeth can position them outside the labial alveolar plate. This can subsequently lead to dehiscence formation.

Miller's Classification of Recession

Whilst many classifications of gingival recession are used in epidemiological research, Miller's classification is probably the most widely used clinical index (Table 9-1). This classification gives the dental surgeon a useful indication of difficulty and potential success of surgical treatment.

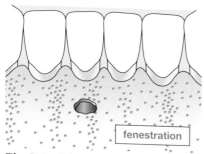

Fig 9-1a Schematic diagram of bony fenestration.

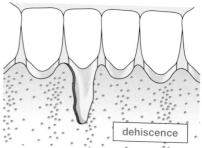

Fig 9-1b Schematic diagram of bony dehiscence.

Table 9-1 **Miller's classification of recession**

Class I: Marginal tissue recession not extending to the mucogingival junction. No loss of interdental bone or soft tissue.	
Class II: Marginal tissue recession extends to or beyond the mucogingival junction. No loss of interdental bone or soft tissue.	
Class III: Marginal tissue recession extends to or beyond the mucogingival junction. Loss of interdental bone or soft tissue is apical to the cementoenamel junction but coronal to the extent of the marginal tissue recession.	
Class IV: Marginal tissue recession extends beyond the mucogingival junction. Loss of interdental bone extends to a level apical to the extent of the marginal tissue recession.	

Management of Gingival Recession

Presurgical Management

Therapy should be directed at plaque control, debridement of any calculus, reduction of inflammation and correction of deficient restorations. Advice should be given regarding an atraumatic brushing technique. Study models or scaled photographs may be used to check for progression of the recession defect.

Presurgical management is a vital first stage in all patients with recession. It is ill-advised and potentially deleterious to carry out surgery in patients whose plaque control methods are inadequate or continue to be traumatic. Where anatomical concerns, such as a prominent fraenal attachment, make plaque control difficult or impossible, however, this should be addressed surgically in the first instance.

The traditional dogma concerning an adequate width of attached gingiva for prevention of attachment loss is not scientifically supported. The health of the gingivae can be maintained independent of their dimensions. There is evidence from both experimental and clinical studies that, in the presence of plaque, areas with a narrow zone of attached gingiva possess the same "resistance" to continuous attachment loss as teeth with a wide zone of attached gingivae (Dorfman, 1982).

Indications for Surgical Intervention

All the indications listed below assume a high level of plaque control and patient motivation:

- Poor aesthetics – the appearance of recession may be unacceptable to the patient, especially if there is an unfavourable high lip line, if teeth appear abnormally long or if gingival margins are irregular.
- Hypersensitivity that cannot be managed with desensitising agents.
- Unfavourable contour of the gingival margin that limits efficient plaque removal.
- Progression of the recession defect.
- Orthodontic tooth movement likely to cause an alveolar bone dehiscence – an increase in the thickness of the covering soft tissue may reduce the risk for development of soft tissue recession.
- Creation of a more favourable soft tissue bed pre-implant surgery (Chapter 11).

Box 9-1 shows contraindications to microgingival surgery.

Box 9-1 **Contraindications to mucogingival surgery**

- Current smoking
- Periodontal pocketing
- Unrealistic patient expectations
- Inadequate connective tissue at donor site
- Severe recession defect – Miller Class IV
- Self-inflicted recession defects
- Prominent fraenal attachments that may need correcting prior to surgery
- Medical contraindications, e.g. patients with scleroderma

Mucogingival surgery is defined as a periodontal surgical procedure designed to correct defects in the morphology, position and/or amount of gingiva surrounding the teeth. The treatment aims of mucogingival surgery are to obtain an increased zone of keratinised tissue and root coverage. There are several different treatment approaches to cover the exposed root:

- free gingival graft
- subepithelial connective tissue graft
- laterally positioned pedicle flap
- coronally positioned flap
- guided tissue regeneration (Chapter 5).

Case Selection and Outcome-related Factors

Mucogingival surgery is a technically demanding procedure that involves delicate manipulation of the periodontal tissues. Mastering these techniques requires training and experience. Careful case selection and choice of procedure are essential to maximise root surface coverage. The following factors should be considered:

- The height of the interproximal bone and interdental papilla influence anticipated root coverage. Root coverage will never extend to beyond the level of the interproximal tissue. In cases where there is bone or soft tissue loss interdentally, the outcome of root coverage is not predictable. Only partial coverage is expected for Class III Miller recession defects, and Class IV recession defects are not amenable to coverage.
- Coverage of a shallow, narrow recession defect is generally more predictable than coverage of a wider defect. Graft survival is highly dependent upon the underlying vascular bed. Wide areas of denuded root surfaces therefore present a host site with minimal blood supply. It follows that covering the root surfaces of molars and prominent canines may be less successful.

- Grafts should not be placed over restorations as coverage will not be achieved. Shallow restorations may be removed prior to grafting.
- Assessment of adjacent soft tissue with regard to the amount of keratinised gingiva is required. This will dictate what type of surgical procedure is chosen for defect coverage.
- The graft must be of an ample size and thickness to cover the denuded area. There is an increased chance of necrosis of the graft where graft tissue is thin or indeed too thick for full revascularisation.
- Post-operatively, close adaptation of the graft with sutures to the recipient site will encourage stabilisation and immobilisation.
- It has been shown that a positive smoking status has a negative impact on periodontal healing following surgery and may lead to failure of root coverage.

Preparatory Treatment

Prominent labial fraena can impede adequate plaque control. A fraenectomy may be considered prior to graft surgery or indeed combined with the graft procedure. This procedure involves severing the attachment of the fraenum to the gingiva. Healing is usually uneventful; however, if a fraenectomy is carried out prior to graft surgery it is sensible to wait for complete healing (Figs 9-2a–d).

Root Preparation

Roots are mechanically prepared prior to any mucogingival procedure to allow biological attachment of the grafted tissue to it. The root surface is thoroughly debrided with ultrasonic or hand instruments and irrigated with sterile saline. The recipient site should be free of plaque and calculus and present a smooth, clean surface.

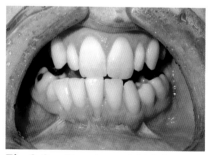

Fig 9-2a Prominent labial fraenum lower central incisor.

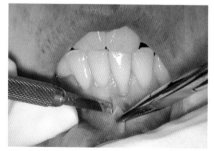

Fig 9-2b Excision of fraenal attachment.

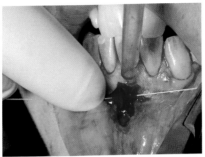

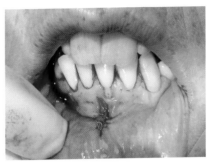

Fig 9-2c Closure with resorbable sutures.

Fig 9-2d Sutured site.

Surgery

There are several different types of mucogingival grafting procedure. This chapter will describe the more popular techniques. Surgical procedures may be divided into two broad categories:

1. *Free Soft Tissue Graft Procedures* – soft tissues are transferred from an area distant to the recession to cover the defect:
- free gingival graft
- subepithelial connective tissue graft.

2. *Pedicle Soft Tissue Graft Procedures* – these types of graft remain attached at their base and involve the positioning of soft tissue over the recession defect; they retain their own blood supply during their transfer to a new location. Examples include:
- Rotational flap procedures including laterally positioned flap and double papilla repositioned flap.
- Flap advancement procedures including coronally repositioned flap.
- Guided tissue regeneration procedures.

Free Soft Tissue Graft Procedures
Free gingival grafts
The free gingival graft has few associated surgical risks and can be utilised to:
- increase the width of the patient's band of keratinised gingiva (e.g. pre-implant)
- prevent reattachment of a high fraenum
- cover exposed roots
- deepen the vestibule.

The technique involves incision at the mucogingival junction at the site of the recession defect, to raise a split-thickness flap and expose underlying connective tissue that must be extended at least 3 mm beyond the recession defect. The thickness of the graft includes palatal epithelium and connective tissue, and optimal thickness is 2 mm. The graft is secured with interrupted sutures and the donor site may also be sutured to stabilise the blood clot. A sequence illustrating this method is shown in Chapter 11 for improving the soft tissue bed around implants.

Subepithelial connective tissue graft
This was initially described by Langer and Langer (1985). This graft is used in a similar way to the free gingival graft. A split-thickness flap (with or without two vertical relieving incisions) is created at the recipient site. The donor connective tissue graft is harvested from the palate using a "trap door" technique. The donor site is usually from the first premolar to first molar region of the palate, avoiding selection of rugae. When harvesting palatal tissue, care must be taken to avoid the greater palatine foramen, thus avoiding the risks of bleeding, paraesthesia and, in the worst case, necrosis of palatal tissues. Any palatal incisions should therefore terminate distally at the mesial aspect of the first molar tooth.

At the recipient site, the split-thickness flap is then sutured over the top of the graft (Figs 9-3a–j; figures adapted from Sato, *Periodontal Surgery: A Clinical Atlas*, 2000). One advantage of this method is that there is a dual blood supply at the recipient site from the subepithelial tissue base and the overlying flap.

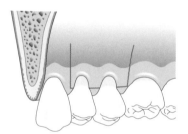

Fig 9-3a Recession defects buccal to maxillary left premolars.

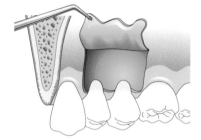

Fig 9-3b Split-thickness flap raised (by sharp dissection).

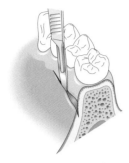

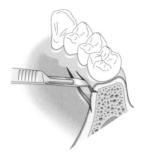

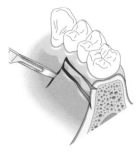

Fig 9-3c Donor site – first horizontal incision is shallow and just through epithelium and surface connective tissue.

Fig 9-3d Donor site – second horizontal incision is down to bone (supraperiosteal).

Fig 9-3e Vertical "trap door" incisions are down to bone (supraperiosteal).

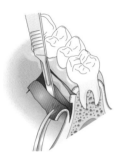

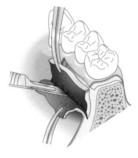

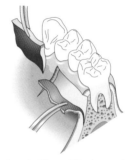

Fig 9-3f Trap door is raised by sharp dissection.

Fig 9-3g Connective tissue graft is dissected free by sharp dissection beneath the graft.

Fig 9-3h Horizontal incision needed at the apex of the connective tissue tail to release graft.

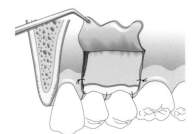

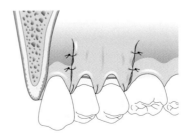

Fig 9-3i Graft positioned over defect.

Fig 9-3j Graft sutured into place.

There are several modifications of this technique that have been described in the literature. The most popular of these include:

- envelope technique (Raetzke, 1985)
- supraperiosteal envelope technique (Allen, 1994a,b)
- tunnel approach (Zabalegui et al., 1999)
- subpedicle approach (Nelson, 1987)
- bilateral pedicle flap tunnel technique (Blanes and Allen, 1999).

A clinical case of a subepithelial connective tissue graft using the supraperiosteal envelope method is shown in Figs 9-4a–g.

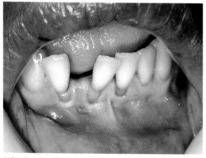

Fig 9-4a Preoperative view of recession defect.

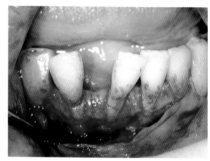

Fig 9-4b Preparation of recipient site.

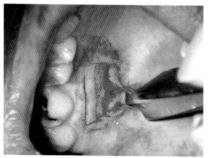

Fig 9-4c Preparation of donor site – trap door approach.

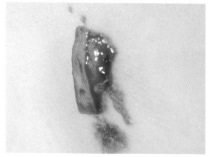

Fig 9-4d Connective tissue graft.

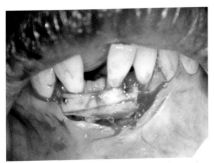

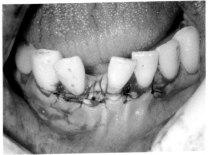

Fig 9-4e Graft sutured to recipient site with resorbable sutures.

Fig 9-4f Split-thickness flap replaced and sutured over the graft.

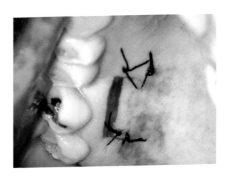

Fig 9-4g Closure at donor site.

Pedicle Soft-tissue Graft Procedures

Double-papilla repositioned flap

The papillae are slid from adjacent teeth and sutured together to cover the defect. Two partial-thickness flaps are prepared that include adjacent papillae. The papillae to be used, when joined together, must have sufficient width and height to cover the defect (Figs 9-5a–b).

Coronally positioned flap

This flap is often used in combination with GTR procedures. A mucoperiosteal flap is raised and the periosteum relieved to allow displacement of the flap. This involves one or two small scores on the underside of the flap through the periosteum. This releases tension in the flap and allows it to be stretched coronally over the defects (Figs 9-6a–c). A resorbable membrane is usually placed beneath the flap to cover the recession defect. The flap is sutured in a new and more coronal position. The technique requires sufficient keratinised tissue apical to the recession defect.

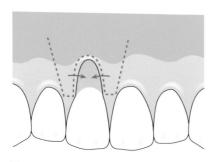

Fig 9-5a Incisions for double-papilla repositioned flap.

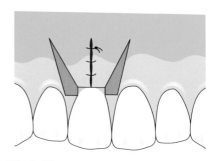

Fig 9-5b Joining of papillae to cover defect.

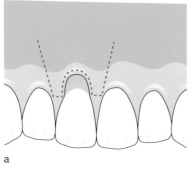

a

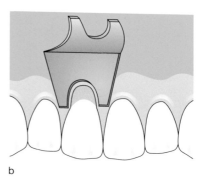

b

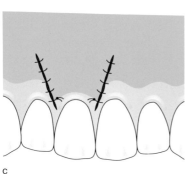

c

Fig 9-6 (a,b) Incisions for coronally positioned flap; (c) Final position of flap.

Table 9-2 gives an overview of the commonly used mucogingival grafting procedures.

Table 9-2 **Overview of commonly used mucogingival grafting procedures**

Technique	Advantages	Disadvantages
Free gingival graft	• Simple • Good for patients lacking adequate vestibular depth	• Second operative site • Donor site leaves large wound • Poor colour match
Subepithelial connective tissue graft	• Dual blood supply • Good root coverage • Suitable for wider recession defects • Small wound at donor site	• Second operative site • Technically demanding – graft is difficult to harvest
Laterally positioned flap	• Intact blood supply of donor tissue • One surgical site • Relatively easy procedure	• Need adequate keratinised tissue at adjacent site • Coverage limited to 1-2 teeth • Danger of gingival recession at donor site
Double-papilla repositioned flap	• Minimal exposure of underlying periodontium • Less tension of donor tissue • One surgical site	• Technically demanding • Poor predictability
GTR used with the coronally positioned flap	• Possibility of enhanced bone formation • Intact blood supply of donor tissue • One surgical site	• Increased cost • Technically demanding • Increased risk of infection

Post-operative Instructions

Patients should be advised to:
- use 0.2% chlorhexidine gluconate twice daily for three weeks as a mouthrinse
- avoid tooth-brushing in the graft area for one to two weeks
- adopt a soft diet
- take analgesics to control pain and discomfort.

Creeping Attachment

Some root coverage may continue to occur by creeping attachment – the post-operative movement of the gingival margin in a coronal direction over areas of a previously exposed root surface. This usually occurs between one and 12 months after surgery.

Assessing Outcomes

It is important to review grafting procedures and maintain a careful audit of outcomes.

Sutures should be removed from the donor site at around one week post-operatively and the recipient site examined gently and carefully for stability. No attempt should be made to remove resorbable sutures from the recipient site.

A review at one month post-operatively will reveal initial healing and should demonstrate root coverage. Further reviews at three months and one year should reveal the full extent of healing and the aesthetic gingival contour (Fig 9-7a,b).

It is normal to observe some shrinkage of the donor tissue in grafting procedures. The experienced surgeon may anticipate this and select a graft size initially to provide greater coverage than may seem necessary. After full healing, consideration may be given to secondary recontouring of tissue for aesthetic reasons where appropriate.

It is unrealistic to expect full coverage of recession defects in all cases, and often partial coverage of the denuded root or increased thickness of tissue (and hence resistance to trauma) may represent a successful outcome.

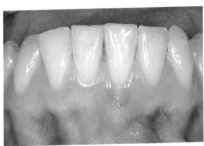

Fig 9-7a Localised recession defect.

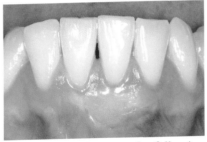

Fig 9-7b Twelve months following treatment with a connective tissue graft.

Complete root coverage has been defined based on the following criteria:
- The marginal tissue reaches the level of the cementoenamel junction.
- Clinical attachment is present.
- Sulcus depth is 2 mm or less.
- Bleeding on probing is absent.

Key Points

- Mucogingival surgery may be considered in the management of localised recession defects.
- Careful case selection and surgical management are critical if a successful outcome is to be achieved.
- In general practice it should be possible to provide initial non-surgical management of recession defects and fraenectomy where appropriate.
- Grafting procedures require delicate, meticulous tissue-handling and further training should be undertaken before these are attempted.
- Where mucogingival surgery is beyond the scope of general practice the practitioner should be aware of cases that are appropriate for referral and the limitations of available treatment options.

References

Allen AL. Use of the supraperiosteal envelope in soft tissue grafting for root coverage. I. Rationale and technique. Int J Periodontics Restorative Dent 1994a;14(3): 216–227.

Allen AL. Use of the supraperiosteal envelope in soft tissue grafting for root coverage. II. Clinical results. Int J Periodontics Restorative Dent 1994b;14(4):302–315.

Blanes RJ, Allen EP. The bilateral pedicle flap-tunnel technique: a new approach to cover connective tissue grafts. Int J Periodontics Restorative Dent 1999;19(5):471–479.

Dorfman HS, Kennedy JE, Bird WC. Longitudinal evaluation of free autogenous gingival grafts. A four year report. J Periodontol 1982;53(6):349–352.

Langer B, Langer L. Subepithelial connective tissue graft technique for root coverage. J Periodontol 1985;56(12):715–720.

Nelson SW. The subpedicle connective tissue graft. A bilaminar reconstructive procedure for the coverage of denuded root surfaces. J Periodontol 1987;58(2):95–102.

Raetzke PB. Covering localized areas of root exposure employing the "envelope" technique. J Periodontol 1985;56(7):397–402.

Zabalegui I, Sicilia A, Cambra J, Gil J, Sanz M. Treatment of multiple adjacent gingival recessions with the tunnel subepithelial connective tissue graft: a clinical report. Int J Periodontics Restorative Dent 1999;19(2):199–206.

Chapter 10
Hard Tissue Surgery (Ridge Augmentation) for Dental Implants

Aim

The aim of this chapter is to outline the role of bone augmentation procedures in relation to dental implant placement.

Outcome

Having read this chapter the reader will be aware of the need for implant placement to be planned from a restorative perspective and when surgical bone augmentation may be utilised to provide predictable results.

Introduction

Traditionally the site of dental implant placement was determined by the location of available bone, and this frequently resulted in sub-optimal implant positioning. Implant treatment planning should be carefully integrated into a holistic restorative plan in order to obtain an acceptable final result. Thought should therefore be given at the initial planning stage to both the prosthetic and the surgical aspects of implant therapy. Surgeons have traditionally either relied on basic surgical stents or placed implants by free hand; however, both methods make it difficult to visualise the final restorative result. Optimal implant position and angulation are crucial to successful restoration, and errors of as little as 1 mm in position or 5° in angulation can significantly and adversely affect the final restoration.

It is common for patients to present for implant reconstruction several years after the loss of their dentition, and the resultant alveolar bone loss presents a major problem for fixture placement. Similarly, the progression of periodontal disease and traumatic injury may result in both tooth loss and loss of supporting hard and soft tissues. When the quantity and quality of bone is inadequate, bone augmentation procedures facilitate reconstruction of the alveolar ridge, allowing for optimal placement and anchorage of implant fixtures.

Various systems have been employed over the years to classify the deficient alveolar ridge, including that of Lekholm and Zarb (1985), Cawood and Howell (1998) and Palacci and Ericsson (2001). The management of deficient alveolar ridges particularly in the anterior maxilla presents a challenge to the surgeon and prosthodontist.

A variety of bone-grafting materials have been advocated and the evidence base for success at five years appears to be satisfactory. The "gold standard" material for bone grafting remains the autogenous bone graft, although the use of allogenic and alloplastic materials is still cited in the literature (Chapter 5).

Autogenous bone grafts can be harvested from several sites (Table 10-1). The major advantages of such grafts appear to be their high osteogenic and osteoinductive potential and rapid conversion to vital bone. Autogenous bone grafts are applied using either an onlay or inlay technique, using either block (Figs 10-1 and 10-2) or particulate grafting techniques. One of the potential problems, as outlined at the planning stage, is that when there is inadequate bone there is often inadequate soft tissue, in terms of both quantity and quality, to cover the graft. This frequently necessitates the need for peri-implant soft tissue augmentation procedures (Chapter 11). However, soft tissue surgery is not a substitute for inadequate hard tissue management around dental implants (Chapter 11).

Table 10-1 **Autogenous bone donor sites**

Extra-oral sites	Intra-oral sites
Iliac crest (Fig 10-10)	Chin
Calvaria	Lateral ramus of mandible
	Coronoid process
	Maxillary tuberosity

Operative Management

Bone Augmentation Procedures for the Anterior Maxilla
Bone augmentation of the anterior maxilla is complicated by the requirement for both aesthetics and function in this area. Although particulate grafts can sometimes be used, in conjunction or not with rigid or resorbable membranes, this provides generally less predictable outcomes compared with the use of cortico-cancellous block grafts (Fig 10-3). The graft of choice in

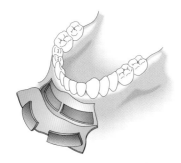

Fig 10-1 Block graft from chin (Courtesy of Palacci, *Esthetic Dentistry*).

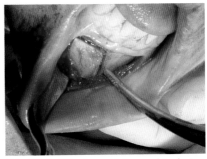

Fig 10-2 Block graft from chin being harvested.

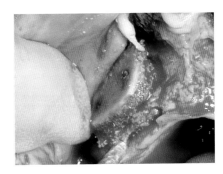

Fig 10-3 Block graft for veneer augmentation to anterior maxilla.

this region is often dependent on the volume of bone required; the more bone necessary, the greater the need for block grafting. Anterior maxillary grafting often necessitates the use of both horizontal and, occasionally, vertical augmentation procedures.

Four techniques are commonly described:
- Veneer grafts – used for horizontal defects.
- Onlay grafts – for vertical defects.
- Split ridge or sandwich technique – for either horizontal or vertical defects.
- "J" or saddle grafts – for both horizontal and vertical defects.

These are demonstrated in Figs 10-4 to 10-7 (based on figures in Palacci, *Esthetic Dentistry*). When placing a veneer graft it is often useful to prepare the recipient bed in a manner similar to a tooth veneer preparation. Taking a thin preparation off the outer buccal cortical plate allows for:

- Better location of the cortico-cancellous block.
- A freshly cut bone surface, thereby creating vascular channels to the cancellous graft, may be approximated.
- A neater adaptation of the graft to the recipient site.

Onlay grafts are less popular because of their unpredictable nature and frequently require preparation of the recipient site to allow for adequate adaptation. Like all autogenous bone grafts (but onlay grafts in particular), rigid fixation is essential to ensure good bone union and healing.

Sandwich graft techniques require the ridge to be split either horizontally or vertically to allow the positioning of an interstitial graft. Sandwich graft techniques (particularly horizontal grafts) are no longer the treatment modality of choice owing to the unpredictable nature of results.

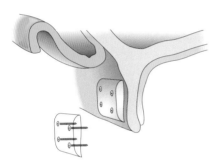

Fig 10-4 Veneer graft.

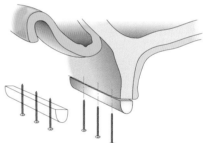

Fig 10-5 Onlay graft.

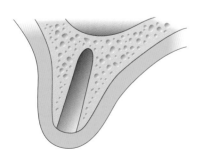

Fig 10-6 Sandwich technique.

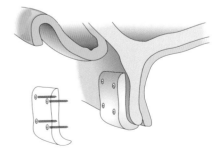

Fig 10-7 "J" graft.

"J" grafts are technically demanding and are commonly sourced from the lower border of the mandible. These grafts have found less favour with some surgeons, who quote surgical morbidity from the donor site as a principal reason for this; however, some institutions quote high levels of success, and it appears that this form of autogenous graft is extremely technique-sensitive.

It is essential with all these techniques that the block graft is rigidly fixed and contoured appropriately for the recipient bed. In addition, soft tissue closure without tension is important to minimise resorption of the grafted material. Often up to 20% of onlay/veneer/"J" grafts may be lost by the uncovering stage three months later; however, this percentage is likely to increase if the overlying soft tissue is under tension or if the graft becomes infected.

Bone Augmentation Procedures for the Posterior Maxilla

Bone loss in the posterior maxilla tends to be in a vertical dimension owing to the orientation of masticatory forces in relation to the occlusal plane. The pneumatisation of the maxillary sinus with age and loss of dentition further contributes to this loss in height. Therefore the onlay and inlay techniques previously described are commonly used. When marked vertical bone loss has arisen, onlay bone grafting is the technique of choice provided that the opposing dentition has not over-erupted (Fig 10-8). This allows for the re-establishment of the occlusal plane without the use of long transmucosal connectors. If minimal vertical height has been lost but the depth of the ridge has been reduced owing to pneumatisation, then a sinus lift inlay graft is indicated (Fig 10-9). Because of the poor blood supply to this region, the use of autogenous bone particulate grafts as opposed to block grafts or alloplastic materials is recommended (Chapter 5). Fig 10-10 shows a graft being harvested. There is still much debate in the literature about the most

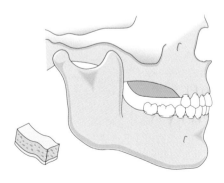

Fig 10-8 A posterior onlay graft (Courtesy of Palacci, *Esthetic Dentistry*).

predictable surgical approaches, the time period for which the graft is allowed to consolidate and the percentage of autogenous bone used in sinus lift procedures. Many authors still advocate the use of 50% autogenous bone particulate mixed with 50% allogenic bone.

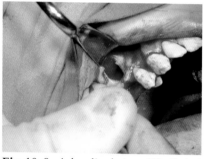
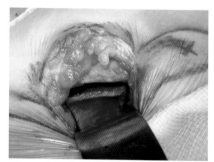

Fig 10-9 A localised sinus lift clinical procedure for an inlay graft.

Fig 10-10 Iliac crest graft being harvested.

Bone Augmentation Procedures for the Mandible

It is often possible, depending on mandibular bone architecture, to shape the residual ridge to facilitate fixture placement by reducing the crest, without the need for augmentation procedures. However, this resective approach is not always suitable because of the residual mandibular dentition or anatomy of the area. In such cases veneer, onlay and split ridge techniques can be utilised. As the cortical bone is most dense in the mandible, it is essential that bone perforation of the recipient site is performed to increase the creation of vascular channels to the graft.

Factors Affecting Success

As with all dental surgical procedures, the success of the operation is dependent on a number of factors, some of which are outlined in Table 10-2 (Buser, 2004). Clearly, many of these factors can be influenced by the clinician or indeed by patient choice, and therefore the correct treatment plan must be appropriate to the individual patient as well as the skill and surgical repertoire of the treating clinician. Ambitious plans undertaken by inadequately trained clinicians for an inappropriate patient will yield either poor results, high morbidity or failure.

Table 10-2 **Factors affecting implant success (Buser, 2004)**

Clinician	Patient	Treatment approach	Implant system
Skills	Medical factors	Evidence-based	Clinical trials
Experience	Dental factors	Risk level	Documentation
Judgement	Anatomical factors and smoking status	Difficulty level	Characteristics

In summary, the dental surgeon must have a comprehensive understanding of the factors outlined in Table 10-2, must make an accurate diagnosis, and must utilise the correct surgical technique to achieve optimal results in the management of osseous defects. The ultimate goal of bone augmentation procedures in relation to dental implant placement is to optimise the aesthetic and functional results of the final implant-borne restoration. Therefore the correct augmentation procedure must be selected to maximise enhancement of the soft tissue profile and the gingival architecture. The average healing time for such an autogenous bone graft for dental implant placement is between three and six months, and complications are often a result of inadequate fixation, infection or inadequate soft tissue closure.

Two questions should always be addressed when considering a bone augmentation procedure:
• Is the procedure technically possible and will it ultimately benefit the patient in terms of their dental implant treatment?
• Is the procedure safe, with minimal morbidity from the donor site, and will it provide a lasting functional and mechanical success at the recipient site?

If the answer is yes to both of these questions then the use of bone augmentation will benefit the definitive implant restoration.

Key Points

• Autogenous bone can be harvested from numerous intra- and extra-oral sites.

- Optimal implant placement is achieved by utilising bone augmentation procedures to replace missing alveolar bone.
- Rigid fixation of bone graft and adequate soft tissue coverage are essential for the success of grafting procedures.
- Bone augmentation, like implant placement, has numerous factors that affect the clinical outcome.

References

Buser D, Martin W, Belser UC. Optimizing esthetics for implant restorations in the anterior maxilla: anatomic and surgical considerations. Int J Oral Maxillofac Implants 2004;19 Suppl:43–61.

Cawood JI and Howell RA. A classification of the edentulous jaws. Int J Oral Maxillofac Surg 1988;17(4):232–236.

Lekholm U and Zarb GA. Patient selection and preparation. In: Brånemark PI, Zarb GA, Albrektsson T (eds). Tissue-integrated prostheses. Osseointegration in clinical dentistry. Chicago: Quintessence, 1985:199–209.

Palacci P, Ericsson I. Esthetic implant dentistry, soft and hard tissue management. Chicago: Quintessence, 2001:137–158.

Further Reading

Hobkirk J, Watson RM, Searson L. Introducing dental implants. Churchill Livingstone, 2003.

Palmer RM, Smith BJ, Howe LC, Palmer PJ. Implants in clinical dentistry. Taylor and Francis, 2002.

Chapter 11
Soft Tissue Surgery Around Dental Implants

Aim

This chapter aims to provide a broad overview of the soft tissue surgical procedures that can be undertaken around dental implants and at what stage in the implant treatment they may be performed.

Outcome

Having read this chapter the reader will be aware of the factors influencing peri-implant soft tissues and will understand the use of techniques designed to improve the quality and distribution of peri-implant soft tissue as well as the timings of such procedures.

Introduction

Dental implants are now well established as part of the dental surgeon's armamentarium for the management of missing teeth and are frequently the most suitable long-term replacement. Whilst there are many different designs of dental implants in terms of surface geometry, surface topography and prosthetic connections, the process of osseointegration is predictable and most implant systems demonstrate high levels of success in well-planned cases. There has been a shift, therefore, in recent years away from osseointegration *per se* towards soft tissue integration and improvements especially in aesthetic areas, although many clinicians are also realising the importance of robust peri-implant soft tissues in non-aesthetic areas.

Peri-implant Soft Tissue Characteristics

The soft tissues surrounding dental implants vary in thickness and level of keratinisation. This in turn affects their appearance and their resistance to oral hygiene measures, and may also affect their long-term positional stability. An implant surrounded by thick keratinised immobile soft tissue is illustrated in Fig 11-1a, whereas Fig 11-1b shows an implant surrounded mainly by thin mobile inflamed non-keratinised mucosa. There is evidence to suggest that non-keratinised mobile tissue around implants has a greater potential

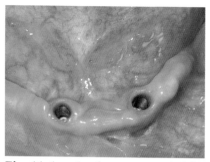 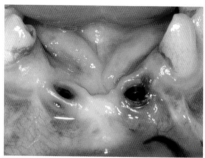

Fig 11-1a Implant surrounded by immobile keratinised mucosa with no evidence of inflammation.

Fig 11-1b An implant with inflamed mobile labial alveolar mucosa.

for inflammation and this *may* be one of several factors that contribute to the long-term success or failure of such implants, particularly in the edentulous setting. Patient comfort during oral hygiene procedures can also be affected by the quality of the surrounding soft tissue and may be a reason for surgical intervention to make the tissue more robust.

Implants Do Not Have a Periodontal Ligament
There are subtle differences between the periodontal gingival soft tissues and those surrounding restored implants. Fundamentally, implants lack a periodontal ligament and the associated blood supply, and this affects the delicate "bundle bone" that lines the coronal part of the socket. The lack of a periodontal blood supply also means that the soft tissues around restored implants have a reduced blood supply compared with natural teeth. This has implications for peri-implant surgical techniques, and the need for meticulous surgical technique is thus paramount. In addition, "late" mucogingival techniques around implants to correct resulting soft tissue problems can be more difficult to undertake successfully than techniques undertaken prior to the final restoration of the implant. Every effort should be made to ensure that the quality/quantity of soft tissues is considered at the time of initial implant treatment and that any soft tissue surgery is planned as thoroughly as any bone surgery undertaken to allow successful implant placement.

Circular fibres predominate around implants, with no evidence of the horizontal inserting fibres that are found in abundance around teeth. This results in a very elastic "cuff" of tissue around the implant, although there is evidence of hemi-desmosomal attachment to some implant abutment surfaces.

Implant Components Affect Soft Tissue Behaviour

The components used to restore implants have effects on the peri-implant soft tissues. Every time a healing abutment is removed and replaced, micro-ulceration occurs and bleeding is generated on removal. Epithelial remnants on the surface of the abutment, if not removed prior to its repositioning, prevent re-attachment of the soft tissues via hemidesmosomes and this results in the epithelialisation of the inner layer of the peri-implant soft tissues. It is also clear that repeated removal and replacement of components at the fixture head level result in the development of inflammation, which can trigger crestal bone loss. The peri-implant soft tissues prefer materials such as titanium, ceramics and zirconium and seem to be able to form a good attachment to them. In contrast, cast gold alloys and plastic materials are not as biocompatible.

Soft Tissue Quality

High quality peri-implant tissues have the following characteristics:
- immobile
- keratinised with good height and width
- good colour match to the surrounding tissues
- absence of inflammation.

The quality of the surrounding soft tissues is dependent on a number of factors but is largely defined by the pre-existing state of the soft tissues at implant placement. This is mainly genetically determined and is referred to as the gingival biotype. Box 11-1 lists some of the factors that may influence peri-implant soft tissue quality.

Box 11-1 **Factors affecting peri-implant soft tissue quality**

- Hereditary gingival biotype
- Number of teeth missing
- Time since extraction
- Previous periodontal inflammation at the site
- Previous flap surgery to the tooth prior to removal
  - Gingivectomy
  - Periradicular surgery
  - Surgery to address resorptive root lesions
- Pre-implant bone grafting procedures
- Implant surgery

Whilst the hereditary gingival biotype is an important factor in predetermining the thickness, degree of keratinisation and scalloping, previous flap surgery related to teeth as well as implant-related surgeries (such as buccal advancement flaps to cover autogenous pre-implant bone grafts or localised GBR, will all tend to reduce the quality of the soft tissues at the implant site.

Previous surgery often produces a degree of fibrous scarring, reduces the blood supply to the marginal tissues and may result in the coronal advancement of the mucogingival line towards the crest of the alveolus, bringing non-keratinised mobile alveolar mucosa with it.

There is also a tendency, several years after tooth extraction, for the gingival remnant to reduce with time to a very thin strip of keratinised tissue over the crest of the ridge, and in some cases this keratinised tissue can disappear altogether.

Mucogingival Procedures Around Implants

The requirement for mucogingival surgery at any given implant site will vary depending on the pre-existing soft tissue status and the requirements of the clinical situation to improve the soft tissue profile for patient comfort or for aesthetic reasons. Essentially, surgery is undertaken for one or more of the following reasons:

* To facilitate the exposure of a two-stage implant.
* To improve the quality of peri-implant mucosa from a thin mobile non-keratinised type to a more keratinised and immobile mucosa.
* To increase the depth of the labial sulcus to improve access for oral hygiene measures.
* To improve the quantity/thickness of peri-implant mucosa in order to correct a thin gingival biotype and as a result achieve a potentially more stable and aesthetic peri-implant mucosa.

In many cases the soft tissue procedure may address more than one of the above, and this is certainly true in the anterior maxilla where peri-implant bone grafting has been undertaken in conjunction with a submerged implant placement, especially in a patient with a thin biotype and a high lip-line. Soft tissue surgery is not, however, a substitute for adequate hard tissue management around dental implants; generally, soft tissues will only be stable if adequately supported by bone.

Types of Peri-implant Surgical Procedures

Many of the peri-implant techniques have been adapted from the mucogingival techniques used around teeth (see Chapter 9). The techniques used can be broadly classified into three groups:

- Free soft tissue grafts:
  - epithelialised graft (free gingival graft)
  - connective tissue graft.
- Local peri-implant soft tissue pedicled flap procedures.
- A combination of free soft tissue graft and local peri-implant pedicled flap technique.

Timing of Surgical Procedures Around Implants

Whilst implant treatment can often be accomplished in a single surgical stage with good results, more complex clinical situations often require a staged approach to treatment with multiple surgical steps.

Peri-implant soft tissue procedures can be undertaken:
- prior to implant placement
- at the time of implant placement
- prior to second stage implant surgery
- at second stage implant surgery
- around restored implants with problems (late procedures).

A number of cases are presented below to illustrate the use of various surgical techniques at different time points within implant treatment.

Free Epithelialised Soft Tissue Graft

Free soft tissue grafts are of use to augment the peri-implant mucosa and are effective in producing an increased volume of soft tissue at the surgical site. Epithelialised grafts are very effective at providing soft tissue of increased keratinisation which is bound down to the underlying bone. This can be very useful when dealing with a shallow labial sulcus and tissue of poor quality (Fig 11-2a–e).

This grafting technique can be used either prior to implant placement, at second stage surgery or as a late procedure following restoration of the implant(s). It is easier to perform prior to implant placement as the graft(s) are easier to immobilise onto a vascularised bed and there is no need to work around the implant abutments.

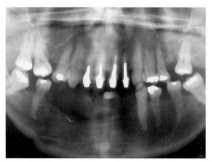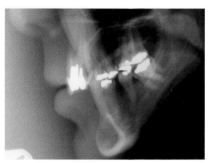

Fig 11-2a Radiographs of a patient with an anterior mandibular edentulous saddle following a road traffic accident 20 years previously.

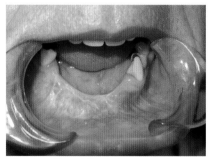

Fig 11-2b Clinical view showing shallow labial vestibule and poor-quality scarred alveolar mucosa.

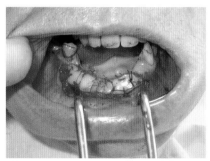

Fig 11-2c Post-surgical view following split-thickness vestibuloplasty and placement of two free keratinised grafts with multiple interrupted and over-sutures.

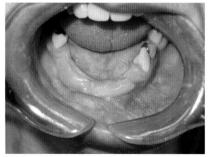

Fig 11-2d Graft incorporation and vestibular deepening six weeks post surgery.

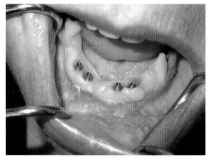

Fig 11-2e Definitive abutments surrounded by thick robust keratinised soft tissues.

Recipient Site Preparation

A split-thickness dissection should be performed, ensuring that the periosteum is left attached to the bone surface and that muscle fibres are removed. The depth of dissection needs to allow for a graft of at least 5 mm width as considerable shrinkage occurs during the maturation phase. The overlying non-keratinised tissue flap can be either removed or sutured down to the apical periosteum.

Epithelialised Graft Harvest from Hard Palate (Fig 11-3a–d)

- Local anaesthesia to harvest site.
- Form a template (from sterile suture packet) to define the size of graft required.
- Place template onto palate or edentulous area, keeping away from the gingival margins of the teeth by 2–3 mm and also avoiding the greater palatine region.

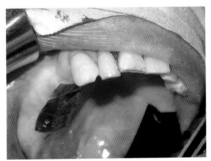

Fig 11-3a Foil template placed at site of keratinised graft harvest.

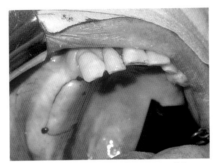

Fig 11-3b Outline of proposed keratinised graft.

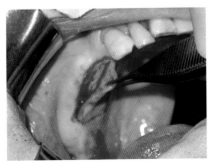

Fig 11-3c Careful dissection is required to obtain a graft of even thickness.

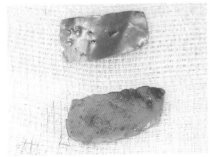

Fig 11-3d Good size match between harvested graft and foil template.

- Using the template as a guide, make a shallow incision around the template just deep enough to score the epithelium and make the incision line bleed.
- Remove the template and begin to harvest the graft by deepening the incisions, trying to keep the scalpel blade at right angles to the mucosa.
- Start to raise the edge of the graft closest to the teeth using a 15 blade, cutting at about 45° until a depth of 1.75–2.00 mm is reached and the edge of the graft can be held by fine forceps.
- Continue to raise the graft, keeping the blade as parallel to the epithelial surface as possible and trying to keep the thickness of the graft as even as possible.
- Complete the final release of the graft and place it into a saline dampened gauze. Apply pressure to the graft site using gauze to reduce any bleeding, although a small ooze often continues despite pressure.
- Protect the site, either using a dressing plate relined with Coe-Pak periodontal dressing or suturing a piece of Surgicel into the site.

Graft Modification

Following removal from the palate, the graft will require a degree of modification before insetting to the recipient site. Any thick areas of the graft containing any fat can be trimmed using a pair of curved scissors (Fig 11-3e), to produce a graft of as even a thickness as possible. The edges of the graft should also be trimmed to remove any bevelled remnants of epithelium and to ensure that the graft has square margins that will allow a good butt joint to be made at the recipient site.

Insetting the Graft

The graft should then be inset at the recipient site using a combination of interrupted sutures and "over-sutures" (Fig 11-2c). The graft should be stretched as much as possible by the marginal sutures, which can be anchored

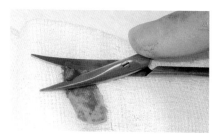

Fig 11-3e Graft modification using curved scissors.

to the neighbouring attached gingivae or to the local periosteum that has been left on the bone by the sharp split-thickness dissection carried out to create the recipient bed. At the end of the procedure, the graft should be firmly immobilised by the suturing and any movement of the lip should not cause movement of the graft. No periodontal dressing to the recipient site is normally required.

Grafting at Second Stage Surgery

At second stage surgery, the grafting procedure must be accomplished together with exposure of the implants. The free grafts need to be trimmed to fit around the abutments and must be positioned so that the majority of the graft is sitting on the prepared periosteal bed. A case in which this technique has been used and which shows the degree to which these grafts contract over time as maturation occurs is illustrated in Fig 11-4a–d.

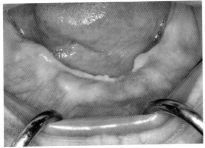

Fig 11-4a Buried implants with overlying thin alveolar mucosa.

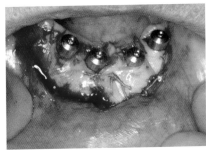

Fig 11-4b Adaptation of free keratinised grafts around healing abutments at second stage surgery.

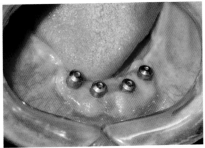

Fig 11-4c Graft appearance at six weeks post surgery.

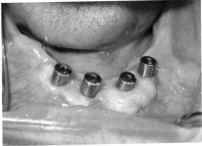

Fig 11-4d Graft appearance at one year post surgery following significant maturation.

175

Late Procedures

Keratinised grafting can be undertaken for late soft tissue implant problems. The use of a free keratinised graft to improve the tissue quality around a previously exposed implant is illustrated in Fig 11-5a–c.

Preoperatively (Fig 11-1b) the peri-implant soft tissue profile was poor and required augmentation to improve patient comfort on cleaning. A free keratinised graft was harvested from the soft tissue tuberosity distal to the upper second molar by a single sweep with a curved 12 blade from distal to mesial, leaving a raw base that healed by secondary intention. The graft was immobilised with multiple over-sutures prior to the application of sustained pressure for ten minutes to ensure good graft adhesion to the underlying recipient bed.

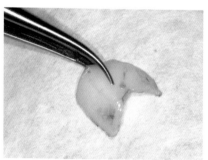

Fig 11-5a Keratinised graft harvested from the soft tissue over the tuberosity distal to the upper second molar.

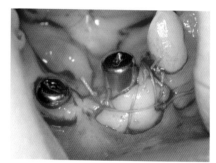

Fig 11-5b Immobilised graft *in situ*.

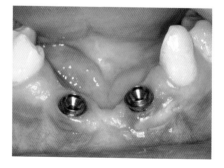

Fig 11-5c Clinical situation three months later showing improvement in the peri-implant soft tissues.

Free Connective Tissue Grafts

The harvesting technique for connective tissue grafts (CTGs) has been discussed in Chapter 9. CTGs are used mainly to increase the thickness of the peri-implant mucosa although they also result in some increase in keratinisation of the overlying epithelium. In contrast to the free epithelialised grafts, CTGs are much more aesthetic and do not change the colour of the gingivae significantly following their use.

CTGs can be used at different time points during implant treatment, always with the basic aim of providing more tissue bulk especially in the anterior maxillary region, where aesthetics are critical. They can be applied at the same time as pre-implant block grafting procedures, at implant placement, prior to and at second stage surgery, or as a late procedure. Most commonly they are applied at implant placement and second stage surgery. Their use at the time of block grafting is often limited by the degree to which the tissues can be mobilised to cover the bone graft and it adds further time and possible complication to such a procedure.

If combined with a two-stage implant placement or as a separate procedure prior to second stage surgery, the procedure is very predictable as the graft is completely buried beneath the overlying flap and the graft can be positioned to augment both the labial aspect and the crestal area. This augmentation of the crestal area is much more difficult to obtain when a CTG is combined with abutment connection.

Once harvested, the CTG is ideally placed directly onto the retained periosteum at the surgical site although it can be placed directly onto alveolar bone or indeed onto membranes. Adequate dissection is required to create the space to accommodate the graft, which should be immobilised with resorbable sutures prior to the final repositioning of the overlying flap at the implant site. The use of two separate connective tissue grafts in a lateral incisor region to provide more soft tissue bulk in a patient with a very high lip line is shown in Figs 11-6a,b.

Local Peri-implant Flap Procedures

The most commonly used soft tissue procedures are local flap procedures undertaken at the time of one-stage implant placement or at second-stage implant surgery and these are summarised in Box 11-2.

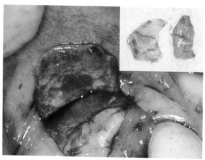

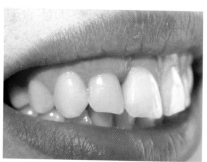

Fig 11-6a Soft tissue augmentation with two separate connective tissue grafts prior to second stage surgery to improve the labial and crestal soft tissue bulk in a lateral incisor region.

Fig 11-6b A good aesthetic result in a patient with a very high lip line.

Box 11-2 **Peri-implant soft tissue procedures**

- At implant placement
    - adaptation of coronal soft tissues around healing abutment or provisional crown (immediate implant placement)
    - roll-flap technique
    - papilla preservation technique (Palacci, 1995)
    - semi-submerged healing
- At implant exposure
    - simple tissue adaptation around healing abutment
    - tissue punch exposure
    - palatal "U" flap
    - papilla preservation technique (Palacci, 1995)
    - roll-flap technique

Simple Flap Adaptation
The simplest local soft tissue procedure is flap adaptation around either a healing abutment or a prosthetic abutment and provisional crown. An example of this, involving a one-stage implant placement in the upper canine region, is shown in Fig 11-7. This was undertaken as an immediate procedure with the extraction of the deciduous canine tooth. In the immediate placement setting this is very straightforward, as the soft tissue architecture is supported by the abutment.

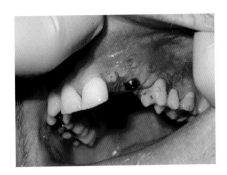

Fig 11-7 Simple flap adaptation immediately following a one-stage implant placement in the upper left canine region.

Semi-submerged Healing

Short healing abutments or specially modified healing abutments with a labial bevel (Fig 11-8) can be placed at implant placement or second-stage surgery in a semi-submerged manner. This allows for some labial gingival overgrowth over the abutment, which produces excess tissue that can be subsequently supported and moulded by application of healing abutments or provisional restorations. This is a useful technique when a significant angulation correction is required and a conventional abutment placed on the implant axis would possibly cause labial recession due to its positioning.

Tissue Punch Exposure

The use of a tissue punch, whilst simple, requires the site to have adequate soft tissue volume present as this technique removes tissue from the implant site. The tissue punch should be used carefully, especially in the aesthetic zone, to remove a core of gingival tissue overlying the cover screw to allow abutment connection. The use of a tissue punch to expose two implants in

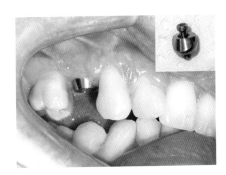

Fig 11-8 Semi-submerged healing with a labially bevelled healing abutment.

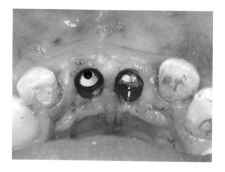

Fig 11-9 Tissue punch exposure of maxillary central incisor implants ensuring preservation of buccal keratinised tissue volume.

the maxillary central incisor region is illustrated in Fig 11-9. The preservation of adequate labial soft tissue volume is achieved by keeping the tissue punch towards the palatal side of the ridge and by using the healing abutment to push the remaining tissues labially.

Palatal "U" Flap Exposure

This is a variant on the tissue punch exposure but without removing any tissue. A palatally based "U"-shaped finger flap is raised to give access to the implant cover screw whilst preserving the interproximal papillae. Once the implant has been exposed and an abutment placed, the flap can be shortened and sutured into position (Fig 11-10).

Papilla Creation Technique

This technique was first described by Palacci (1995) and was designed to help form interproximal papillae between implants at first or second stage implant surgery. The initial crestal incision is to the palatal aspect of the ridge and is full thickness, with mesial and distal relieving incisions (Fig 11-11).

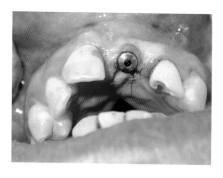

Fig 11-10 Exposure of a central incisor implant via a palatal "U"-shaped finger flap.

180

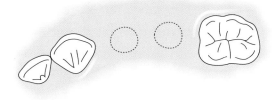

Fig 11-11a
Situation prior to
second stage surgery
with outline of implants
shown.

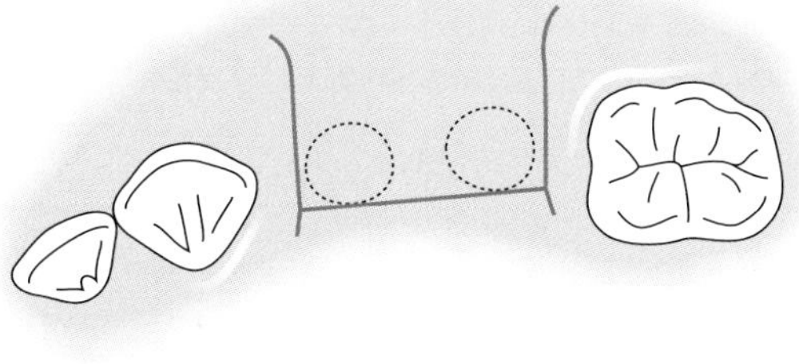

a

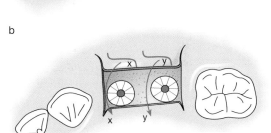

Fig 11-11b
Full-thickness crestal
incision at the palatal
line angle of the
implants with buccal
and short palatal
relieving incisions.

b

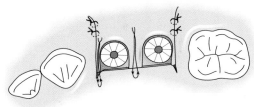

Fig 11-11c
Following abutment
connection, S-shaped
incisions are made to
create interdental soft
tissue pedicles which lie
passively in the inter-
proximal spaces.

c

Fig 11-11d
Soft tissue closure with
a combination of
interrupted and "over-
sutures" over the pedicle
flaps.

d

Once the healing abutments are placed, small semi-lunar bevelled incisions are made from distal to mesial, creating small fingers of tissue, which are turned into the interdental areas between the healing abutments. Sutures are placed over the delicate pedicle flaps to hold them in position during healing and to reduce the vascular compromise that might occur by suturing directly through them.

The Roll Flap

The roll flap is a full-thickness buccally placed flap, which incorporates a palatal connective tissue "tail" that can be rolled beneath the buccal flap to augment the buccal soft tissue volume in the cervical region. This can be undertaken for a one-stage implant placement or at implant exposure (Fig 11-12). A split-thickness crestal incision is made just to the palatal side of the ridge and is continued palatally for 5–6 mm to create a connective tissue tail which is attached to the main flap. The connective tissue is released from the underlying bone by further incisions and with the use of a periosteal elevator. Once the combined flap is raised, the connective tissue part is rolled beneath the main buccal flap, which is sutured in place around the healing abutment. Often a small palatal defect remains following the raising of this flap, which heals by secondary intention.

Key Points

- Soft tissue surgery around implants is helpful to improve the quality of the peri-implant tissues, which may help with aesthetics and oral hygiene measures.
- Soft tissue surgery is not a replacement for adequate hard tissue management.
- Free keratinised grafts require preparation following harvest and need to be well immobilised at the recipient site.
- Free connective tissue grafts are a useful adjunct in aesthetic implant therapy to improve soft tissue thickness.

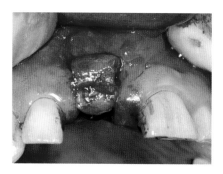

Fig 11-12 A roll flap with connective tissue tail prior to tucking the connective tissue beneath the buccal flap.

References

Palacci P. Peri-implant soft tissue management: papilla regeneration technique. In: Palacci P, Ericsson I, Engstrand P, Rangert B (eds). Optimal implant positioning and soft tissue management for the Branemark system. Chicago: Quintessence, 1995:59–70.

Further Reading

Sclar A. Soft tissue and esthetic considerations in implant therapy. Carol Stream IL: Quintessence, 2003.

Index

Quintessentials for General Dental Practitioners Series

in 50 volumes

Editor-in-Chief: Professor Nairn H F Wilson

The Quintessentials for General Dental Practitioners Series covers basic principles and key issues in all aspects of modern dental medicine. Each book can be read as a stand-alone volume or in conjunction with other books in the series.

Publication date,
approximately

Clinical Practice, Editor: Nairn Wilson

Culturally Sensitive Oral Healthcare	available
Dental Erosion	available
Special Care Dentistry	available
Evidence Based Dentistry	Autumn 2007
Infection Control for the Dental Team	Winter 2007
Therapeutics and Medical Emergencies in the	Winter 2007
Everyday Clinical Practice of Dentistry	

Oral Surgery and Oral Medicine, Editor: John G Meechan

Practical Dental Local Anaesthesia	available
Practical Oral Medicine	available
Practical Conscious Sedation	available
Minor Oral Surgery in Dental Practice	available

Imaging, Editor: Keith Horner

Interpreting Dental Radiographs	available
Panoramic Radiology	available
21st Century Dental Imaging	available

Periodontology, Editor: Iain L C Chapple

Understanding Periodontal Diseases: Assessment and Diagnostic Procedures in Practice	available
Decision-Making for the Periodontal Team	available
Successful Periodontal Therapy – A Non-Surgical Approach	available
Periodontal Management of Children, Adolescents and Young Adults	available
Periodontal Medicine: A Window on the Body	available
Contemporary Periodontal Surgery – An Illustrated Guide to the Art Behind the Science	available

Endodontics, Editor: John M Whitworth

Rational Root Canal Treatment in Practice	available
Managing Endodontic Failure in Practice	available
Adhesive Restoration of Endodontically Treated Teeth	available

Prosthodontics, Editor: P Finbarr Allen

Teeth for Life for Older Adults	available
Complete Dentures – from Planning to Problem Solving	available
Removable Partial Dentures	available
Fixed Prosthodontics in Dental Practice	available
Occlusion: A Theoretical and Team Approach	Autumn 2007
Managing Orofacial Pain in Practice	Winter 2007

Operative Dentistry, Editor: Paul A Brunton

Decision-Making in Operative Dentistry	available
Aesthetic Dentistry	available
Communicating in Dental Practice	available
Indirect Restorations	available
Dental Bleaching	available
Choosing and Using Dental Materials	Autumn 2007
Composite Restorations in Posterior Teeth	Winter 2007

Paediatric Dentistry/Orthodontics, Editor: Marie Therese Hosey

Child Taming: How to Manage Children in Dental Practice	available
Paediatric Cariology	available
Treatment Planning for the Developing Dentition	available
Managing Dental Trauma in Practice	available

General Dentistry and Practice Management, Editor: Raj Rattan

The Business of Dentistry	available
Risk Management in General Dental Practice	available
Quality Matters: From Clinical Care to Customer Service	available
Practice Management for the Dental Team	Winter 2007

Dental Team, Editor: Mabel Slater

Team Players in Dentistry	Winter 2007

Implantology, Editor: Lloyd J Searson

Implantology in General Dental Practice	available

Quintessence Publishing Co. Ltd., London

Polymeric carbons –
carbon fibre, glass and char

RENEWALS

You may phone to renew this book twice on 01429 857173. Please note we are unable to renew books which are overdue or reserved by another borrower.